Other Voices

While we have made enormous progress in the HIV response in many countries, we are not on track to end AIDS. Barstow's book shows the critical juncture the global community faces in turning the tide on the epidemic. Barstow's message is both startling and clear: we must act now to reboot and recharge our efforts to deliver sustainable results for people and communities across the world.

—**Professor Peter Piot**
   Director, London School of Hygiene & Tropical Medicine
   Founding Executive Director, UNAIDS

David Barstow's book is a must read for anyone who cares about the world's collective conscience and future. In creative and compelling fashion Barstow presents the stark choice and moral imperative that confronts us to not only reverse the HIV and AIDS crisis but to end it.

—**Rev. Adam Taylor**
   Executive Director, Sojourners
   Author, *Mobilizing Hope: Faith-Inspired Activism*
   for a Post–Civil Rights Generation

The HIV response has been one of the most successful in the history of public health. If we act now, we can get to the end. If we do not, history will not treat current policy makers well.

—**Amb. Mark Dybul**
   Professor of Medicine, Georgetown University
   Co-Director, Center for Global Health and Quality
   Former Executive Director, The Global Fund to Fight AIDS,
   Tuberculosis and Malaria

(Continued on the next page)

The World Council of Churches supports David Barstow's book *HIV and AIDS in 2030: A Choice Between Two Futures* and has chosen the future where the faith community remains faithful to ending HIV and AIDS because it is a moral and Biblical imperative. Accordingly, the World Council of Churches reaffirms the theological foundation of the Church as a healing community that was verbalised in the 1986 Executive Committee statement "AIDS and the Churches"; recommits to the 2016 Pastoral Letter "Churches Recommit to Accelerate HIV Response;" recommits to playing an active and leading role in ending HIV and AIDS; urges churches, faith communities and other religious institutions to likewise recommit to playing their parts in ending HIV and AIDS, keeping the presence, lived experience and participation of people living with HIV central in their ministries. Finally, the World Council of Churches urges the world's leaders to strengthen the global response and funding to ensure that HIV and AIDS are eliminated as threats to public health by 2030.

—**Prof. Dr. Isabel Apawo Phiri**
 Deputy General Secretary: Public Witness and Diakonia,
 World Council of Churches

If we needed a wake up call, here it is. *Two Futures* smacks its readers with the mirror Barstow wants us all to face, asking everyone to own up to her role in finally ending AIDS. And the legacy of HIV ultimately will have a ripple effect across multiple global health responses modeled after this success story, not only those affected by the disease and their allies. You have been warned.

—**Loyce Pace, MPH**
 President and Executive Director, Global Health Council

In 2001, when World Vision was ramping up its AIDS prevention initiatives, I called HIV a "Doomsday Virus"; the kind of apocalyptic pathogen that is the stuff of disaster movies. It stalked its prey silently, passed from husband to wife and mother to child, showed no symptoms for months or even years so that it could continue to be transmitted unnoticed, and was effectively 100% fatal. To make it worse, because it was spread through sexual contact, it became taboo to even discuss it openly. Only a full-court press by the nations of the world could stop it. And, remarkably, the world responded and began to win the battle to raise awareness, slow its spread and care for its victims. But HIV, like a wolf at our door, doesn't give up. David Barstow's book lays out two possible storylines based on the two possible choices the world might make. One is the "Doomsday" scenario of terrible human suffering, and the other is the victorious ending where humanity 'wins' and the threat is averted. We can write this next chapter, but what will we write? The choice is ours to make.

—Richard Stearns
  President Emeritus, World Vision US

The next decade will truly decide if we will end this epidemic in the U.S. and everywhere. It is a public health, public policy, and human rights imperative that Barstow knows well.

—Jesse Milan, Jr.
  President and CEO, AIDS United

We've made a commitment to bringing HIV and AIDS under control by 2030, and we know how. Not to do so is a policy choice—and a policy failure—with tragic consequences.

—Amb. Jimmy Kolker
  Former Chief of HIV/AIDS Section, UNICEF

(Continued on the next page)

In search for why and how the evolution of HIV/AIDS epidemic could take a better turn?

Two Futures provides sobering insights into the unintended effects of global action and inaction in addressing the HIV/AIDS epidemic. By the effective use of anecdotes, fiction and imageries, David paints a paradoxical picture of avoidable regrets for past inactions/missed opportunities, and the potential positive returns on focused investments in achieving the HIV/AIDS 95-95-95 goals by 2030

David portrays the present and future perspectives in provocative tone, highlighting barriers to be overcome and opportunities to be leveraged in addressing the HIV/AIDS epidemic. Over the years, due to several impactful initiatives aided by close intimacy with communities, faith-based/inspired organizations/networks have been frontline actors and innovators in making sustainable progress in achieving HIV/AIDS goals in sub-Saharan Africa. Hence, the Author's gracious recognition of the indispensable role and positive influence of faith-based leadership and religious assets in changing the HIV/AIDS trajectory should serve as an impetus for faith-inspired organizations/ networks, especially in sub-Saharan Africa.

In many ways, David Barstow's book represents the much-awaited prophetic voice of global conscience, convening forum and advocacy platform for global collective action towards ending the HIV/AIDS epidemic with the fierce urgency of now!

—Peter Yeboah
    Chairman/President,
    Africa Christian Health Associations Platform

Dr David Barstow has been unrelenting in his fight against HIV and AIDS related stigma and discrimination. In his book, *HIV and AIDS in 2030: A Choice Between Two Futures,* he outlines the two possible trajectories. We, as faith communities, have a choice. We can win the battle if we stand and work together towards a future without AIDS. A future without AIDS is possible!!

—**Rev. Phumizile Mabizela**

   Executive Director, INERELA+, International Network of Religious Leaders Living with or Personally Affected by HIV or AIDS

David Barstow imagines two futures: one where we succeed, and one where we do not. Success means saving millions of lives and will only happen if governments, civil society and the extensive faith community networks work together to mobilize policy and resources to bring HIV under control. We must keep our eye on the ball …

—**Doug Fountain**

   Executive Director, Christian Connections for International Health

We must return to the sense of urgency and recharge our efforts. Barstow makes it clear the heavy price the world will pay for not doing so.

—**Dr. Michael Merson**

   Professor of Global Health, Duke University

   Author, *The AIDS Pandemic: Searching for a Global Response*

(Continued on the next page)

Thanks to a remarkable global effort, and the advocacy led by people living with HIV, we have made tremendous progress against HIV and AIDS. The end is in sight and we know how to get there. But as Barstow makes clear, we will only get there if we choose to do so and if we persist to the end. Faith leaders and communities are crucial to that choice and to that persistence.

— **Jacek Tyszko, UNAIDS Senior Advisor for Faith Engagement**

HIV and AIDS in 2030

HIV and AIDS in 2030

A Choice Between Two Futures

David R. Barstow, PhD

GOYTS Publishing

Design by Meadowlark Publishing Services.
Cover illustration © Shutterstock.com/Yulia Ogneva.
Manufactured in the United States of America.

ISBN 978-1-7331424-0-3

Published by GOYTS Publishing.

Published 2019

This book is dedicated to the many local religious leaders who have had the courage to address the social complexities of HIV and AIDS with love and compassion rather than judgment and rejection.

Contents

Foreword

On a balmy Sunday evening in July, 2000, President Thabo Mbeki of South Africa stood up to warmly welcome 12,000 of us gathered in Durban for the biennial International AIDS Conference. He then proceeded to lay out his AIDS denialism manifesto, claiming that AIDS treatment was a CIA-Big Pharma plot. That manifesto cost nearly a half million South African lives before AIDS activists forced a policy reversal. Today, South Africa has the largest AIDS treatment program in the world.

In *HIV and AIDS in 2030: A Choice Between Two Futures*, Dr. David Barstow returns us to Durban three decades later for the 2030 International AIDS Conference. He provides two parallel transcripts of a plenary panel of government officials, academics, and secular and faith-based NGO leaders. One—set in a future in which AIDS has come back strongly—is a conversation of regret, frustration, disappointment, missed opportunities, and a feeling of failure for having lost the war against AIDS. The other—set in a future in which AIDS is no longer a public health threat—is a conversation of joy, achievement, and great satisfaction over having won the war against AIDS.

Dave and I met in June 2018, when we were asked to lead a

dialogue on ending AIDS at the annual Christian Connections for International Health conference we were both attending. I've since come to greatly respect and admire Dave, who gave up a successful career in academia and business to fight the dehumanizing impact of HIV and AIDS stigma. He attributes that determined shift to a remark by activist/rock star Bono at a 2006 Christian leadership conference.

A self-described "computer scientist turned AIDS activist," Dave deftly combines the meticulous attention to order and detail you would expect from a scientist with the persistence and passion for action you would expect from an activist. The fruits of this combination are evident in *Two Futures.*

Dave's compelling and vivid approach lays out the implications of the choice confronting policy makers, funders, and other world leaders today. He worked closely with modeling experts and drew on published analyses, UNAIDS Fast Track projections, and the Global Fund Investment Case to ensure the win and lose scenarios and charts are plausible, well supported, and based on the latest data.

In human terms, the difference between the two futures couldn't be more chilling: the current 1 million annual AIDS deaths could be reduced to less than 340,000 in the best-case "win" scenario or swell to nearly 1.5 million deaths in the worst-case "loss" scenario.

Is such a resurgence possible? I fear so, especially if "AIDS fatigue" and competing national and international priorities are allowed to undermine the gains from the unprecedented global response to AIDS over the past two decades.

We know how to end AIDS. At the time of AIDS 2000, the range of proven prevention methods was limited, the cost of AIDS medicines was sky high, funding was grossly inadequate, deaths were increasing, and families were on their own to care for the sick and orphaned. Today, we have a wide range of tools and resources for prevention, care, and treatment, from post-exposure and pre-exposure prophylaxis, to established global and national supply systems, to effective approaches tailored to the circumstances of key populations.

The benefits of ending AIDS would be substantial. The dramatic decrease in new cases would especially benefit youth and women, who would suffer the most from a resurgence of AIDS. Reducing new cases and the resulting need for costly lifelong treatment would also contribute to the viability of universal health coverage programs expanding in every region of the world.

Finally, ending AIDS is affordable. Affected low- and middle-income countries are now bearing nearly two-thirds of the burden from public and private funding sources. The remainder comes from governments, foundations, and private sources in the U.S. and other high-income countries. To end AIDS by 2030, an additional $8 billion per year is needed from all sources. Against this increase, economists calculate that ending AIDS will generate economic returns of more than $460 billion.

If the AIDS epidemic has taught us anything, it is that the human and economic cost is huge each time national or world leaders deny, debate, and delay taking action, as President Mbeki did. Yet, as Martin Luther King Jr. reminds us, the greatest threat to social justice is not its opponents but the "appalling silence" of its many supporters.

In *Two Futures*, Dave Barstow makes it clear that we can win the war against AIDS—or lose it. The outcome we reach is not a matter of speculation. It is a matter of choice: to take action or to sit back. It is a choice that rests with our political and public health leaders. It is choice that rests with each of us as global citizens to raise our voices. Ultimately, it is a moral choice for which we have the know-how, the resources, and no excuse for not acting.

—Jonathan D. Quick, MD, MPH

Author, *The End of Epidemics: The Looming Threat to Humanity and How to Stop It*

Adjunct Professor of Global Health,

Duke Global Health Institute

Preface

How could that be? I asked myself as I stared at charts that showed a resurgence of HIV and AIDS in the 2020s. Surely, we're on track to end AIDS, maybe slower than we'd like, but do these charts mean it might actually come back in the future? After all the great progress we've made, we might still lose?

It was the fall of 2015. I was in New York City at a meeting about the global response to the AIDS epidemic. Somebody from the United Nations was presenting quantitative models of the future of the epidemic through the year 2030. In one scenario, HIV and AIDS actually make a resurgence in the 2020s: there would be more new HIV infections and more AIDS-related deaths in 2030 than in 2015. I was caught by surprise. Perhaps I shouldn't have been—I'd been active in the faith-based response to AIDS for almost a decade and had learned a great deal about the epidemic—but I was genuinely shocked that a resurgence of AIDS was a real possibility in the future.

My shock was magnified by the fact that the world already knew how to end the AIDS epidemic. We had treatment options that enabled people living with HIV to live long, productive lives, and we had a variety of techniques to prevent HIV transmission. So, in 2015, we knew what to do to prevent a resurgence in the 2020s and to end HIV and AIDS as public health threats by 2030.

I could not imagine a future in which we didn't do what we knew how to do, but those charts were showing me just such a future. *What would it feel like?* I asked myself. What would it feel like to be in a similar meeting in 2030, where the charts were showing a current reality, not just a future projection? What would it feel like to have witnessed a human catastrophe—a catastrophe that had cost many millions of lives—and to know that we had allowed it to happen, that we could have prevented it, but didn't? What would it feel like to lose the war against AIDS, knowing that we could have won?

I have written this book because losing is not inevitable. There is still time to win the war against AIDS. We have the capability and capacity to create a future similar to a different scenario presented at that meeting in New York, a future in which HIV and AIDS are no longer threats to public health. But it will require an explicit choice, a strong commitment to action and perseverance. The two futures portrayed in this book illustrate our alternatives, highlighting both the ways in which we will make our choice and the human consequences of making it.

In the time since that meeting in New York, we have continued to make great progress in many ways, but the risks of losing the war against AIDS have also increased. The window of time for making the choice to win is closing, but it is not yet closed. It is not too late to choose the future.

David R. Barstow, PhD
June 2019
Corvallis, Oregon, USA

It's not too late to choose a future …
… when HIV and AIDS are no longer global threats

Global commitment to end AIDS

American leadership is vital to maintaining the global commitment to end AIDS by 2030.

Global funding for the AIDS response

Replenishment of the Global Fund in 2019 by donor countries is essential, together with increased funding commitments from recipient countries.

Continued strong funding for PEPFAR is also important, due to the strong leadership role that it plays in the global response to HIV and AIDS.

Universal access to HIV services

HIV services must be available for all who need them, including treatment services for those infected, as well as prevention services for at-risk populations. These services must be provided without judgment, stigma, discrimination, or risk of criminal prosecution.

Stigma and discrimination

Social and political leaders must recognize the health consequences of stigma and discrimination and must take steps to combat them.

Education and empowerment of young people

Prevention programs for young people are vital to prevent a rapid increase in new infections. Youth programs must include education about HIV, AIDS, and all prevention options, as well as supportive social environments.

Innovation in science and medicine

Advancements in science and medicine will enable us to increase the effectiveness of HIV treatment and prevention services.

Policies based on scientific evidence

Policies must be guided by the best available scientific evidence about effectiveness, including treatment and prevention programs focused on the needs of at-risk populations.

Country-specific strategies

Global success depends on national strategies that recognize the risks of HIV and AIDS within their boundaries and provide prevention and treatment programs appropriate to those risks.

It's not too late to choose a future …
… when the HIV epidemic in the United States is over

National commitment to end AIDS in the United States
Many American cities and states are fully committed to ending AIDS. *Ending the HIV Epidemic,* a new program introduced in 2019, represents an opportunity for a national commitment with realistic prospects for elimination of HIV and AIDS as public health threats before 2030.

National funding for the AIDS response
Funding for the *Ending the HIV Epidemic* program is obviously essential. In addition, it will be important to develop, fund, and implement an effective national program to end the opioid epidemic in order to reduce the associated risk of HIV infection.

Universal access to HIV services
Further expansion of Medicaid would help provide treatment services to more Americans living with HIV. In addition, it will be important to ensure that HIV infection is not treated as an exclusionary pre-existing condition by health insurers.
The *Ending the HIV Epidemic* program includes specific HIV prevention services focused on the needs of at-risk populations in certain areas. In addition, it is important that general prevention and testing services be low-cost and easily accessible to all.

Stigma and discrimination
Social and political leaders must recognize the health consequences of stigma and discrimination and must take steps to combat them.

Education and empowerment of young people
Many American young people are dangerously unaware of HIV and AIDS. It is vital that all young people be educated about the full range of prevention options.

Policies based on scientific evidence
Policies for HIV education, prevention, testing, and treatment services must be guided by the best available scientific evidence about effectiveness.

It's not too late to choose a future ...
... when religion is a strong partner in ending AIDS

Religious commitment to end AIDS

Religion has a vital role to play in ending AIDS. Success will require a commitment to advocacy and action. It will require dealing with the social complexities associated with HIV and AIDS in a spirit of love and compassion rather than judgment or rejection. It will require treating all people with dignity and respect, protecting the vulnerable, and reaching out to the marginalized.

Religious leaders

Advocacy by prominent religious leaders, stressing both the moral imperative to end AIDS and the urgency to act now, can serve as a much-needed global conscience.

Advocacy by religious leaders can also help ensure that HIV prevention and treatment services are available to all, without judgment, stigma, discrimination, or risk of criminal prosecution.

Religious communities

Local religious communities can be instrumental in reducing stigma, in supporting adherence to treatment, in educating and empowering young people, in reducing gender-based violence, and in reaching out to the marginalized.

More data about the actions and effects of local religious communities would be very helpful in guiding future religion-based initiatives.

Religion-based organizations

Organizations with a religious motivation or background have long been important providers of HIV services, and they must continue to play this role as long as the epidemic continues.

Strengthened integration with global response

The AIDS response, both globally and domestically, would be stronger and more effective through increased collaboration and coordination between secular and religious initiatives.

HIV and AIDS in 2030

HIV and AIDS in 2030

2030 will be a year of reckoning for the AIDS epidemic, marking fifty years of one of the worst epidemics in the history of the world. The 28th International AIDS Conference, which will be held in July 2030, is likely to be a focal point of world attention. The conference may be held in Durban, South Africa, just as earlier conferences have been held in Durban marking other key points in the global response to AIDS. The conference will probably include a panel of leaders looking back on the fifty-year history of HIV and AIDS. But what will the panelists say?

If HIV and AIDS have made a strong resurgence in the 2020s, the panelists will focus on what went wrong. Perhaps the panel will be called *How We Lost the War Against AIDS*. The panelists will look at charts that show rates of new infections and deaths, first rising, then falling, then rising again. They will look at charts showing treatment coverage, and they will look at charts showing the financial investments that were made and not made. They will remember the great progress made in the 2000s and 2010s. But they will focus their discussion on what went wrong, what led to the tragic resurgence of the AIDS epidemic. They will identify the mistakes that were made and the opportunities that were missed. It will be a very sober discussion, because they will know that the catastrophe could have been avoided.

But in a different future, a future in which HIV and AIDS are no longer threats to public health, the panel will have a joyous tone. Perhaps the panel will be called *How We Won the War Against AIDS*. These panelists will also look at charts of new infections and deaths, treatment coverage, and financial investments, but their charts will all show steady progress toward the end of AIDS. They will look at the key events and key decisions that kept the global progress going, even during times that were politically or socially challenging. They will identify the mistakes that were avoided and the opportunities that were seized. And they will celebrate!

Curiously, or perhaps not so curiously, the two groups of panelists will say very similar things. They will both talk about the importance of global political will and global commitment. They will talk about the complexities of the social issues that affect so much of the AIDS epidemic. And they will talk about the very significant effect that religion had on the epidemic, sometimes in a positive way and sometimes in a negative way.

Although the two groups of panelists will say similar things, they will say them with very different tones. On one panel, they will say them with regret, recognizing challenges that were not overcome. They will face accusatory questions from the audience, spoken with grief and anger. The panelists will share a sense of collective guilt that the world hadn't done what it could have done.

On the other panel, they will say the same things with satisfaction, describing the challenges that had been overcome. They will hear congratulatory comments from the audience, spoken with joy and gratitude. The panelists will share a sense of collective pride that the world had accomplished what some thought would be impossible.

But, of course, it is now only 2019. We don't yet know what the panelists will say, because we don't yet know what future we will give to them. We don't yet know whether we will win or lose the war against AIDS. If we persevere, we can still win. If we do not persevere, we will surely lose. The choice between these two futures is ours to make, and we must make it now.

How We LOST the War Against AIDS

Transcript of a Plenary Session
28th International AIDS Conference
Durban, South Africa
29 July 2030

Note from the Editor

There was an unusually large amount of media coverage of the 2030 International AIDS Conference, recently held in Durban, South Africa. Much of the media coverage was related to one specific panel session and the massive demonstrations that occurred outside the conference center while the panel was being held. Given this heightened interest, members of the Program Committee of the IAC have decided to make publicly available a complete transcript of the panel session. The transcript has been compiled from video recordings of the panel session. The words are those spoken by the panelists and audience members, except for minor edits to improve the flow.

David R. Barstow, Editor
5 August 2030
Corvallis, Oregon, USA

Question from the Audience

You can all see the signs around the edges of the auditorium, the ones that say "YOU LOST THE WAR AGAINST AIDS!" How do those signs make you feel?

Mr. De Jong

For me, it's angry. The world could have won the war, we knew what to do, but we didn't. We blew it! And now a whole lot of people are dead.

Amb. Rogers

Maybe a little bit extra from me would have saved millions of lives. I don't know, but I hate to think I might have made the difference.

Dr. Nkosi

The outcome of the game affected real people leading real lives. For them, it wasn't a game. They are the ones whose feelings really matter.

Imam Karume

Rev. Phumzile Mabizela, the former Executive Director of INERELA+, once said, "If we can't do this, what good are we?" Well, we couldn't do it. We could have done more, we should have done more. But we didn't. So now I ask, what good are we?

Introduction

Dr. González

Could you all please find seats so we can get started. I know there was a lot of commotion and confusion outside the hall, and that has delayed the start of the session. You can all help us get going if you take your seats.

While you are taking your seats, I'd like to update you on the demonstrations that took place throughout Durban today. We believe they are the largest demonstrations in the history of the AIDS epidemic. The police have estimated that over 200,000 people participated. I, for one, am grateful for that. We needed something to draw greater attention to the ongoing AIDS epidemic. I hope that the demonstrations will help.

I also hope that this panel will help. We deliberately gave the panel a provocative title, *How We Lost the War Against AIDS*. None of us really believe we have totally lost the war, although it sometimes feels like it. In fact, some of us are uncomfortable even calling it a war. But it is worth noting that the death toll from AIDS is now close to the death toll from World War II. So even if the fight against AIDS isn't the same kind of war, its effects are just as serious.

It looks like things have settled down in the auditorium. Let's get started.

My name is Dr. Rafael González. It has been an honor to serve as the President of the International AIDS Society for the past two years. In that position, I am one of the Co-Chairs of this conference, the 28th International AIDS Conference.

This is now the third time that the International AIDS Conference has been held in Durban. Each time has marked a significant turning point in the AIDS epidemic.

The 13th IAC was held here in July 2000. It was the first time that the AIDS conference had been held in Africa and marked the global recognition of the magnitude of the AIDS epidemic.

Sixteen years later, the 21st IAC was held here in July 2016. It marked the first time that we believed we might actually be able to end AIDS. We had achieved remarkable progress, really amazing progress, in getting people with HIV on ARV treatment. And there was a strong sense that we had it in our power to end AIDS as a public health threat by 2030.

Now it is 2030, and, as we all know, that optimism was badly misplaced. AIDS is still a public health threat. In fact, with the increasing rates of new HIV infections, the resurgence of AIDS in the 2020s, and the prospect of rising death rates, HIV and AIDS are now perhaps greater threats to public health than they have been at any time since that first Durban AIDS conference thirty years ago.

This panel has been assembled to help us understand what went so tragically wrong. How did we lose the war against AIDS, a war that we fully expected to win?

The panel will be moderated by Dr. Zhang Xiu Ying, the Director-General of the World Health Organization. Dr. Zhang, could you please introduce the other panelists and start the discussion.

Dr. Zhang

Thank you, Dr. González.

So the question is: how did we lose the war against AIDS? We have invited eight panelists with distinguished backgrounds to help us answer this question. On the stage here with me, from your left to your right, we have:

Imam Ahmed Karume, the Executive Director of INERELA+, the International Network of Religious Leaders Living with or Personally Affected by HIV or AIDS.

Dr. Munashe Nkosi, the Executive Director of the Global Fund to Fight AIDS, Tuberculosis and Malaria.

Mr. Joost De Jong, the Executive Director of WHN, the World-wide HIV Network, an advocacy group for people living with HIV.

Rev. Emily Morgan, the Executive Director of Christian Health Alliance, a consortium of Christian NGOs.

Dr. Chibuzo Okafor, the Director of African Projects for International Interfaith Relief Services, a coalition of relief service organizations from a variety of religious traditions.

Dr. Olivia Bennett, the President and Chief Executive Officer of the Campaign to End AIDS in America, a leading AIDS advocacy organization in the United States.

Dr. Jaylen Thomas, the Director of the Centers for Disease Control and Prevention in the United States.

Amb. Christopher Rogers, the United States Global AIDS Coordinator. He runs what we all know as PEPFAR.

You can find more information about our panelists in your printed program.

I should add that the panelists today will be speaking as individuals, not as representatives of the organizations they work for. Opinions they express do not necessarily represent official positions of their organizations.

You may notice that the panelists are primarily public health experts, AIDS activists, and religious leaders. We have several scientists and doctors, but their careers have not focused on research or providing medical services directly to patients. That was a deliberate choice when we planned this panel. We won't be discussing the medical aspects of the epidemic. HIV and AIDS are very complex, but scientists and doctors have figured out the answers. The reason we lost the war against AIDS is not lack of scientific and medical knowledge.

I will start this session by reviewing the basic epidemiological data from the fifty-year history of the AIDS epidemic. Then we will have open discussion among the panelists about three specific topics: funding, social drivers, and religion. In order to stimulate a livelier discussion, I have asked the panelists not to discuss the topics amongst themselves prior to their appearance on this panel. Of course, knowing the panelists as I do, it seems quite likely that they ignored my request!

Following the discussions about the three topics, we will open the panel to questions from the floor. We hope to have about twenty minutes for questions. We will then have brief closing statements by the panelists.

Shall we begin?

Fifty Years of the AIDS Epidemic

Dr. Zhang

You have all seen this chart *[Figure 1, below]* before. It shows the annual rates of new HIV infections and AIDS-related deaths in the fifty years since the epidemic began in 1980. This is worldwide.

To quickly review the data, there was a rapid increase of new infections during the first fifteen years, peaking at 3.4 million in 1995, then a gradual decline in new infections until the end of the 2010s, followed by a moderate increase. The new infection rate appears to have stabilized at about 1.9 million per year.

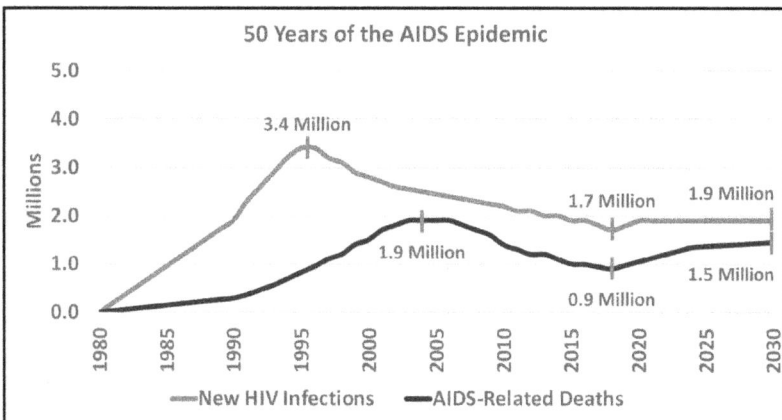

Figure 1—Fifty Years of the AIDS Epidemic

With respect to deaths from AIDS-related causes, there is, of course, a lag behind new infections. The rates rose gradually through the mid 2000s, then declined for about a dozen years, then began increasing again. The lag behind new infections is not as great now as it was in the early days of the epidemic because some of the deaths are people who were on treatment but then went off treatment when the supplies of medications started to run out. The rate of AIDS-related deaths is now about 1.45 million per year, and we hope it has stopped rising.

[Editor's note: At this point, about two dozen demonstrators rose from their seats, raised placards, and started chanting, "YOU LOST THE WAR! YOU LOST THE WAR!"]

Dr. Zhang *[addressing the demonstrators]*
Please take your seats. We understand your anger. We share it! That's why we're having this panel. Please let us continue.

[Editor's note: The shouting lasted for several more minutes while the demonstrators were returning to their seats. Some remained standing around the perimeter, holding placards that said, "YOU LOST THE WAR AGAINST AIDS!"]

Dr. Zhang
Thank you.

To pick up where we left off, we were talking about AIDS-related deaths. During the fifty years of the epidemic, a total of 52.3 million people have died. As Dr. González mentioned, that is actually pretty close to the number of people who died during World War II, which was the deadliest military war that the world has ever experienced. That was actually one of the ideas behind the title of the panel. The war against AIDS has become one of the deadliest wars in human history.

Now in looking at this chart *[Figure 2, below]*, the time when things started to go wrong was near the end of the 2010s. To help understand what happened then, and the implications for the decade of the '20s, here's a chart that shows treatment coverage for the twenty-year period between 2010 and 2030.

As seen on this chart, the number of people living with HIV has grown steadily from thirty-two million to forty-four million. The number of people who know their status grew at a slightly faster rate, then slowed down in the first half of the 2020s, then picked up again. The number on treatment rose quickly through the 2010s, but then started dropping off as the supply of medications began to decline. It has started to rise again during the past five years. The number of people who achieved viral suppression also rose steadily, from five million to about seventeen million in 2019, then dropped and held steady at about thirteen million in the first half of the 2020s, then started rising again to about twenty-four million now.

Most of you recall the Fast Track program, initiated by UNAIDS in 2015 with the goal of quickly gaining control of the epidemic by

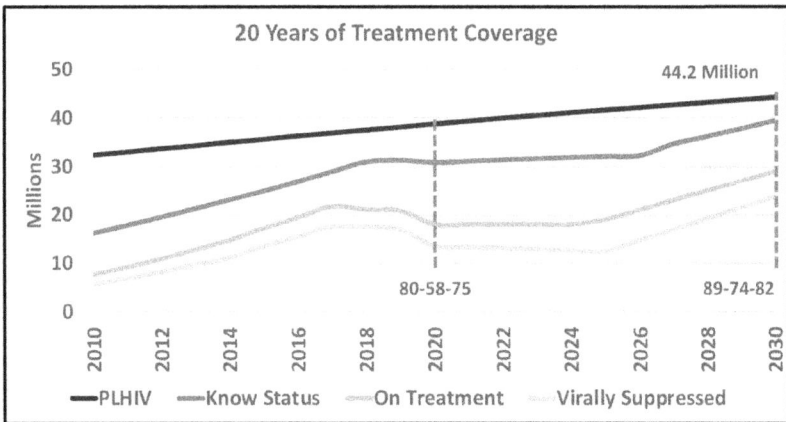

Figure 2—Twenty Years of Treatment Coverage

2020 and then eliminating HIV and AIDS as public health threats by 2030. This was part of that optimistic mood of the 2016 Durban conference. The intermediate goal for 2020 was described as 90-90-90: 90% of people living with HIV know their status, 90% of them are on treatment, and 90% of them have reached viral suppression. As the chart shows, we fell substantially short of the 2020 target, reaching only 80-58-75, which meant that only about a third of people living with HIV had suppressed viral load. So we didn't have anywhere near the preventive effect that widespread viral suppression would have given us.

Here's one more chart [Figure 3, below].

As you know, the ratio of incidence to prevalence has been used for the past decade as a single indicator of epidemic control. A ratio below 0.030 is generally thought to represent control of the epidemic. We were on a steady trajectory downward, with a hope of reaching the threshold seven or eight years ago. But the indicator stopped the downward decline in the late 2010s, rose briefly, and then has gone down slowly. It is currently at 0.043, far short of epidemic control.

Any comments before we go on to the three topics?

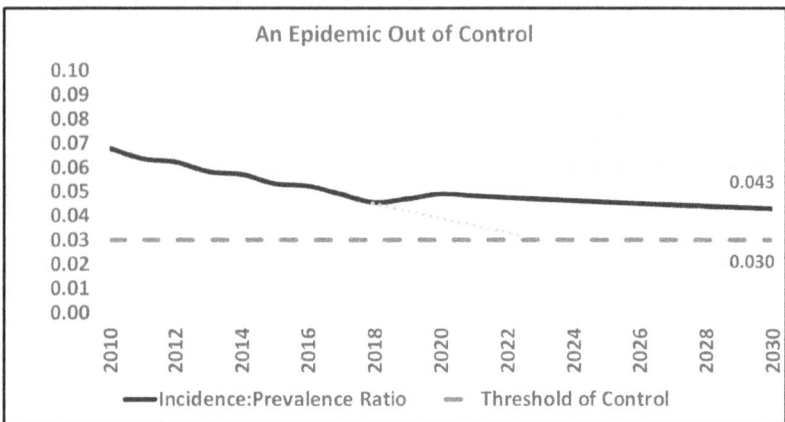

Figure 3—An Epidemic Out of Control

Dr. Okafor

Just one. The thing that really stands out is the line for new infections. Fifteen years ago, we all believed that the rate of new infections would continue to go down. In fact, what was it? 2017, 2018? That's when we first realized that the rate of new infection wasn't going down as fast as we expected, that perhaps we wouldn't get the epidemic under control as quickly as we thought. That was also when we started to realize that the next generation of young people was especially at risk. We certainly saw that in Nigeria, and our worst fears became true. There was a large increase in new infections among our young people in the 2020s.

Dr. Zhang

Yes, you're right about the rate of new infections. One goal of this panel is to better understand why we were wrong, why we didn't slow down the rate of new infections.

Dr. Thomas

Also, remember our hopes for a vaccine? The first one came out in 2024, yet there was no observable effect on new infections. I mean, obviously there was an effect. The vaccine was only 60% effective, but it was still a significant help to people who used it. And we expected it to have a significant effect on the epidemic overall, but on the scale of these charts, it was barely a little blip.

Dr. Zhang

Yes, you're right.

OK, now let's start on our first topic.

Why Did We Reduce Funding for AIDS?

Dr. Zhang

The first topic is money. This chart *[Figure 4, below]* shows the overall global investment in the AIDS response for the past twenty years.

Now this is global investment—the total amount of money spent on the AIDS response worldwide: PEPFAR, Global Fund, internal domestic sources, rich countries, poor countries, foundations, everything. As you can see, it was at $15 billion in 2010, rose for a few years, peaking at about $21.5 billion, and then dropped

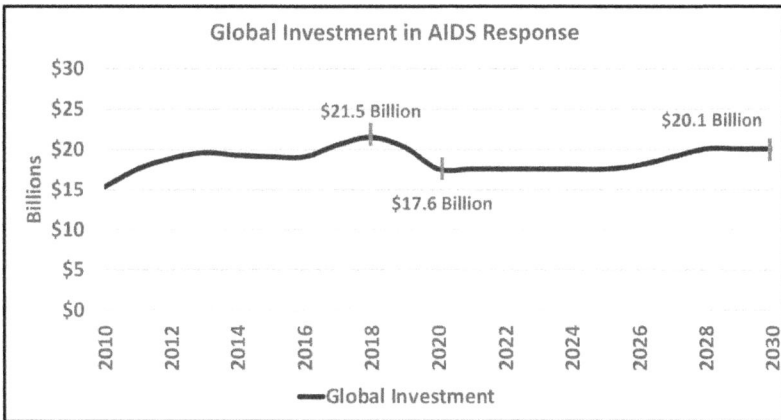

Figure 4—Global Investment in AIDS Response

Dr. Zhang Xiu Ying:
It's safe to say that the drop in global investment in the late 2010s was a major factor that led to the resurgence of HIV and AIDS. There's absolutely no doubt about that.

---

quickly to about $17.6 billion in 2020, a cut of about 18%. It held steady until 2025, when global investment started to rise again.

There's an obvious correlation between this chart and the previous charts. It's safe to say that the drop in global investment at the end of the 2010s was a major factor that led to the resurgence of HIV and AIDS. There's absolutely no doubt about that.

The deeper question is: why was there such a precipitous drop? And, in this case, I think we can very usefully focus on a single event, namely the Global Fund replenishment in 2019. The Global Fund had made its investment case for an increase of about 15%, but instead, the donor nations actually cut investment by 20%. This was quickly followed by cuts in other bilateral programs. The recipient countries were able to make up some of the shortfall, so the overall global investment was reduced by only 18%. Looking back, the replenishment decision was obviously the step that triggered the global reduction. So let's focus on that single event, as representative of global decision making about the AIDS response during those critical years.

So my question for the panelists is: why did we reduce the Global Fund investment in 2019? What do you think?

Dr. Nkosi

Before discussing that, it's important to recognize something you haven't mentioned: the decisions that implementors had to make when faced with funding cuts. What do you cut? Do you cut treatment or do you cut prevention? Prior to that time, the strategy was pretty clear: get as many people as possible on treatment and run good prevention programs. But with the funding cuts, it wasn't so easy. Do you cut back on treatment or do you cut back on prevention? Obviously, treatment, especially reaching viral suppression, is an important part of prevention, but there are other parts, like awareness, education, condom distribution, PrEP, medical male circumcision, even vaccines, that are also important. So the implementors had a real problem. Do you emphasize prevention, reduce treatment, and risk the lives of people living with HIV? Or do you emphasize treatment, reduce prevention, and put future epidemic control at risk?

Dr. Zhang
Thank you, Munashe. That's a really good point. We know that different implementors took different approaches, and we could spend many hours debating which strategy was best. But let's focus today's discussion on what led to the funding cuts, not the effects of the cuts.

Dr. Okafor
OK, first, let's remember that the 2019 Global Fund decision didn't come as a surprise out of nowhere. For several years, there had been signs of a weakening of political will. Remember the 2016 political declaration from the UN High-Level Meeting on AIDS? I was there for that meeting. There was a lot of talk and argument about what the right level of funding should be, a lot of resistance to fully funding the UNAIDS Fast Track program. And then, a few months later, at the 2016 Global Fund replenishment meeting, it was a real struggle to get what we got. So the 2019 decision wasn't a surprise.

Dr. Thomas

You're right, of course, and that reflected a certain amount of what you might call AIDS fatigue. Governments were tired of thinking about AIDS. We certainly saw that in the U.S. And we saw it in the discussions about the Sustainable Development Goals, where AIDS got less emphasis than fifteen years earlier with the Millennium Development Goals. So AIDS fatigue was a part of it.

Amb. Rogers

And related to fatigue was complacency. Many, many people thought that the AIDS crisis was over. Why should we keep pouring money into it? Especially when there were several other issues that became more prominent, like climate change, economic inequality, mass migrations, or even other diseases, like Ebola. AIDS had been a top-level issue in the 2000s, but by the end of the 2010s, by the time of the 2019 Global Fund decision, AIDS had much lower visibility, and governments spent less time and energy on it.

Dr. Nkosi

Fatigue and complacency. That's where I think we really could have used the strong American leadership that had been so vital in the previous decade and a half. Remember, it was President Bush who launched PEPFAR in 2003. That was a remarkable act of American leadership. President Bush saw a huge humanitarian problem and committed the U.S. to solving it. And that strong American leadership continued for the next fifteen years, but it began to weaken in the late 2010s, exactly the period when global funding started to fall. The U.S. could have led the way in overcoming fatigue and complacency.

Dr. Thomas

Wait a minute, it's far too easy to simply blame Americans.

Dr. Nkosi

Oh, I'm not really blaming them. They had done so much good for so long. I just wish they had kept at it a little longer during this rough period.

Mr. De Jong

Back to complacency. You know, it wasn't only complacency. There was also indifference. Complacency means you think things are OK. Indifference is when you don't really care one way or the other. And, sometimes, I think it was even hostility, a feeling of anger that so much money had been spent on people and countries that should have been able to take care of themselves. Remember, this time period we are talking about, the late 2010s, was the high point of the populist and nationalist movements in the U.S. and Europe. And anger and resentment toward other people and other countries and other problems was a big part of that. In fact, that's probably one of the root causes of the weakened American leadership.

Rev. Morgan

You know, in a certain way, the resentment is even understandable. We probably should have expected it. The AIDS crisis was largely seen as rich countries providing all the money and poor countries spending it. That was an oversimplification, of course, and over time, more and more of the financial cost, in fact a large fraction of it, was provided by the high-burden countries themselves. But that took a long time to get started. Think back thirty years ago, to the first Durban AIDS conference, when President Mbeki publicly denied that HIV causes AIDS. That denialism delayed the South African AIDS response by several years. What would have happened if South Africa had responded more aggressively, more quickly? And if South Africa had used the funds more effectively? Then donor countries would have seen that South Africa was doing its part, and it would have been easier to get money both in the early 2000s and in 2019.

Dr. Zhang

Thank you all. Let me see if I can summarize what you have said. The funding cuts at the end of the 2010s were the result of several factors—AIDS fatigue, complacency, or indifference—but it mostly came down to a loss of political will. To some degree, we can attribute that to weakened American leadership, but realistically speaking, there was a lot of blame to go around.

With that, I'd like to move on to our next topic now.

Dr. Bennett

Before you do, I'd like to comment on the situation in the United States. Our model of health care, with its emphasis on private health insurance, was different from many other countries, so it's a little hard to relate to the charts of global funding and the 2019 Global Fund decision. Perhaps the closest analogy was when we tried to expand our publicly funded program called Medicaid in the early 2010s. Many people living with HIV got their treatment through Medicaid. But, unfortunately, many of our states didn't expand Medicaid within their borders. Those decisions, collectively, meant that a lot of people with HIV couldn't afford treatment services. And, of course, there was that moment in 2019 when we launched a new domestic HIV strategy. Unfortunately, that initiative failed because it was too limited to fully control the HIV epidemic in the U.S. In fact, at that time, there were some aspects of health care policies in the U.S. that actually got in the way of ending HIV in the U.S.

Amb. Rogers

I'd like to add one more thing about the funding question. Many of you were here in Durban, in fact in this very hall, in 2016. And if you were, you heard Charlize Theron give an amazing speech. I went back and found the text of her speech. I think she perfectly expressed the real reason that global AIDS funding fell so short of what was needed. Here's what she said:

> *The real reason we haven't beaten the epidemic boils down to one simple fact: We value some lives more than others. We value men more than women. Straight love more than gay love. White skin more than black skin. The rich more than the poor. Adults more than adolescents.*

That's really what it all came down to.

[Editor's note: At this point, there was prolonged applause, lasting several minutes.]

Dr. Nkosi

That's a great quote. And it's interesting to look at in the context of a discussion about investment. We can never tell for sure what might have been, but the estimates I've seen are that the investment reductions at the end of the 2010s ultimately cost between eight and ten million lives. And I'll bet most of those lives were lives that, as Charlize would say, we value less than others. If someone had said in 2019 that our decision would kill eight to ten million of the "more valuable" lives, maybe we would have decided differently.

Dr. Zhang

Thanks, Munashe. That's a sobering thought, and there's probably more truth to it than any of us would like to admit.

And, actually, this makes a good lead-in to the next topic.

How Important Were the Social Issues?

Dr. Zhang

The next topic is about everything except money. Let's suppose that there had been sufficient funds available for the global AIDS response. Let's suppose that the Global Fund replenishment meeting in 2019 had gone the other way, that the donor countries had agreed to the 15% increase that had been requested. And that domestic funding in high-burden countries had been stronger. And let's suppose that other funding decisions around that time had gone in a way that would assure adequate funding. Would that have been enough to ensure that we had eliminated HIV and AIDS as public health threats by now? Or were there other things that we needed to do? To put it succinctly, when we ask how we lost the war against AIDS, was lack of funding the only problem? What do you think?

Amb. Rogers

Let's start by reminding ourselves about what Jonathan Mann said. For those younger people in the audience who don't know who Jonathan Mann was, back about forty years ago, he was the leader of the first WHO AIDS initiative and a vigorous human rights advocate. This is what he said. Actually, I didn't do as well as Chris with Charlize's quote. I didn't find out exactly what words he used, but the essence was this:

AIDS is a social problem…
…with some medical aspects.

His point was that, in many ways, the social drivers were more important than medical issues. And yet, if you look back at where we put our money and energy, we spent just a tiny fraction to address the social drivers. If Jonathan Mann was right, then we were spending all our money on the least important aspects. Look, I know it's much more complicated than that. The medical and scientific work cost a lot, but it produced amazing results, so it was obviously money that was very well spent. But I also know that we should have paid a lot more attention to the social issues a lot earlier.

Dr. Nkosi
Yes, you're right. And I'll bet it would have even been cheaper in the long run. If we had done a better job with the social drivers earlier, then we might not even have needed the increase that the Global Fund was looking for in 2019.

Dr. Zhang
Let me add that we had this in mind when we planned this panel. As I mentioned before, we won't be discussing the medical aspects of the epidemic. We know what to do about HIV and AIDS. And we knew what to do in the late 2010s. The challenge is always what to do with what we know.

Rev. Morgan
Don't forget, there was a point very early in the epidemic when we didn't do the right thing with what we knew. There is a tried-

and-true strategy for dealing with contagious diseases that threaten public health. You identify the people who are infected, trace their contacts to find others who are already infected or potentially exposed, treat everyone, and keep tracing to make sure you contain the epidemic. We could have done that in the early days of the AIDS epidemic, and we would all be a lot better off right now. But we let social issues get in the way.

Amb. Rogers
I think that was Jonathan Mann's whole point. The social issues do get in the way. They make it much harder to follow that strategy. It's very difficult to track people when the people being tracked feel judged and threatened. It can even make things worse by driving them into hiding.

Rev. Morgan
Tracking people doesn't mean judging and threatening. It can be done with dignity and respect and compassion.

Amb. Rogers
Yes, it can, but we didn't do that very well.

Look, let's be specific here about the social drivers. There are some social drivers that cause problems for any epidemic. Poverty, mobile populations, malnutrition, unsanitary water, weak medical delivery systems, incarceration. But there are some social drivers that are specific to HIV and AIDS, mostly because of the modes of transmission. For example, when women have a lower social status than men, they are particularly vulnerable to HIV infection through sexual activity.

Dr. Jaylen Thomas:
We know that the epidemiological effects of stigma are real. We have all sorts of studies that show the effect of stigma.

Mr. De Jong

And, of course, there's stigma. Infection with HIV is associated with activities that are considered bad by large segments of the population, whether it's sex outside of marriage, same-sex relationships, injection drug use, transgender people, sex work. All of those are considered bad in one way or another.

[Editor's note: At this point, about two dozen demonstrators rose from their seats and started walking around silently carrying signs that said, "STIGMA KILLS." This lasted for about five minutes.]

Dr. Zhang *[addressing the demonstrators]*

Please take your seats. Remember, we are on your side. We know that stigma kills. It's been killing for a long time. That's why we're talking about it.

Joost, could you finish your thought, please?

Mr. De Jong

Well, the thought is simple really. When behavior is considered "bad," it leads to judgmental attitudes, stigma, and social isolation. And these, in turn, cause people to avoid testing and treatment.

Dr. Bennett

We certainly saw those effects of stigma in the United States. For example, black gay men were doubly stigmatized, and their rates of HIV infection are astronomical, with HIV prevalence now over 50%.

Dr. Thomas

We know that the epidemiological effects of stigma are real. We have all sorts of studies that show the effect of stigma. We know that fear of being judged by neighbors and fear of rejection by society often stop people from getting tested and treated. We know that stigma decreases a person's sense of self-worth and that a decreased sense of self-worth leads to poor health decisions, not only about testing and treatment, but also about prevention.

Imam Karume

Speaking of personal health decisions, it seems to me that, for a long time, we overemphasized individual personal responsibility for prevention. Remember the ABC strategy first rolled out in Uganda in the late 1990s? For those who don't know about this, the ABC stood for "Abstain, Be faithful, use a Condom." That certainly lays all the blame on the individual, as if society doesn't have any responsibility at all. Personal responsibility is obviously very important, but it's not everything. What about rape and other forms of gender-based violence? Or poverty that forces young girls to choose between two bad alternatives? Or laws that push some groups of people into hiding, where diseases like HIV can thrive?

Mr. De Jong

All of this emphasis on personal responsibility just increases the stigma. Think about what ABC is really saying. "You should abstain from sex, but if you're not a good enough person to abstain, you should at least be faithful to your spouse, and if you can't even do that, then use a condom." In other words, if you use a condom, or even think about using a condom, it's because you have failed to achieve the top two criteria of goodness. You must be a truly bad person.

Mr. Joost De Jong:
Long ago, we identified various populations that were at increased risk of HIV infection. And the thing about them was that many of these populations were somehow outside of mainstream society; they were marginalized.

Dr. Munashe Nkosi:
Some of these populations weren't that far outside the mainstream of society. Like young girls and women, who are so vulnerable in many societies.

Dr. Bennett

In the U.S., this notion of personal responsibility played a role in our debates about health insurance. For many years, we couldn't figure out sensible ways to deal with pre-existing conditions, and I think that some of our difficulty was an unconscious assumption that any pre-existing condition was somehow the fault of the person who had it. And, of course, infection with HIV was seen as an example of a pre-existing condition that resulted from irresponsible personal decisions.

Rev. Morgan

But you can't say that personal responsibility doesn't matter! It is absolutely vital that everyone take responsibility for the things they can control.

Mr. De Jong

No one is saying that personal responsibility doesn't matter. Of course it does, but we also have to make sure that people have tools to exercise that responsibility, and we have to ensure that we have a social context that supports personal responsibility.

Dr. Nkosi

OK, we've talked a lot about stigma, which is basically an attitude. There was also obviously a lot of outright discrimination, discriminatory behavior. We saw a lot of it in health clinics, churches, courts, workplaces. I mean, people were outright fired from work even though being HIV-positive had nothing to do with the job they were doing. We had discrimination all over the place. And, of course, discrimination just reinforces stigma. It proves that people's fears are justified.

Mr. De Jong

Another form of discrimination was travel. For a long time, people were unable to travel to the U.S. and other countries, or they had to interrupt their treatment to be able to travel, which just increased drug resistance. And don't forget criminalization. Many kinds of behavior that were seen as anti-social or against the norm were against the law. Fear of criminal prosecution certainly stopped a lot of people from getting tested for HIV and from accessing prevention services. I know it's not realistic, or even desirable, to change all those laws, but we needed some way for people to get HIV services without being afraid of being thrown in jail.

Dr. Zhang

Yes, I'm sure you're right, Joost. We should have done some things differently. But what? What should we have done differently about the social drivers? If we had paid more attention to what Jonathan Mann said, what would we have done?

Imam Ahmed Karume:
What you are talking about is empowering people to take care of themselves, and empowerment includes education about all the prevention methods.

Imam Karume

Well, for one thing, I think we somehow needed to come to grips with the realities of human behavior. It's a lot more complicated than most of us would like to think. Especially in the early years of the epidemic, there was a lot of wishful thinking about what people are really like.

Mr. De Jong

Also, we somehow had to be better at accepting people's differences. Long ago, we identified various populations that were at increased risk of HIV infection. And the thing about them was that many of these populations were somehow outside of mainstream society; they were marginalized. And the very fact that they were marginalized was part of the problem. As we know, HIV thrives among the marginalized.

Dr. Nkosi

Some of these populations weren't that far outside the mainstream of society. Like young girls and women, who are so vulnerable in so many societies. Of course, if they became infected with HIV, that often led to being marginalized, simply because of the disease.

Dr. Bennett

Wasn't that the point Charlize made back in 2016? That's actually why I think the 2019 initiative in the U.S. collapsed. It included many programs specifically focused on key populations, but, ultimately, as a society, we Americans just weren't ready to do what those populations needed.

Amb. Rogers

Exactly. And, of course, the rest of society forgets that the margins aren't as solid as we might think. Sex workers have clients who also have other sexual relationships and might be married. Women who have been raped hope to lead normal family lives. Recovering injection drug users are trying to fit back into society. Men who have sex with men may sometimes have sex with women. The gaps in the margins are why HIV has become a generalized epidemic in so many places.

Dr. Thomas

Something that would have helped a lot would have been to pay more attention to the scientific data about what works and what doesn't work. For example, the data showed that abstinence-only prevention programs don't work, but we still pushed them for much too long. We also knew that mass distribution of condoms didn't work either, but for a long time, that seemed to be all anybody talked about. Then there is the very strong link between HIV and sexual- and gender-based violence. We did not consider this adequately enough in programming and also did not consider how HIV added to the risk of sexual- and gender-based violence. Or what about needle-exchange programs? We knew they helped prevent HIV transmission, but we were still pretty slow to roll them out. Or criminalization. We knew that criminalization of same-sex behavior led to higher rates of HIV transmission. It took us an awful long time to accept the fact that scientific data often showed that trying to enforce certain kinds of behavior made the epidemic worse rather than better.

Rev. Morgan

You know, there was another way that we didn't use scientific data. The evidence has always been clear that reducing the number of sexual partners reduces the risk of HIV transmission. Yet we somehow seemed reluctant to spread that message. We could have done a much better job of spreading that part of the prevention message.

Imam Karume

What you are talking about is empowering people to take care of themselves, and empowerment includes education about all the prevention methods. ABC was at least a start at personal empowerment, flawed as it might have been. But we really needed much more widespread education early on in the epidemic, both about the nature of HIV and AIDS and about all the various options for preventing HIV transmission.

Dr. Bennett

We certainly saw that in the United States. Not only did we fail to educate people about how to prevent HIV infection, we didn't even teach people what HIV is! I remember giving a talk, ten or fifteen years ago. After the talk, a young woman came up to me and asked, "So what exactly is HIV? I've heard it is some kind of sexually transmitted disease." I was appalled that she knew so little!

Rev. Morgan

We also should have had stronger support systems for individuals, both those with HIV and those at risk of infection. Remember the DREAMS program PEPFAR had in the late 2010s? That did a really good job of helping young girls. I wish PEPFAR had had the funds to keep it going and even to roll it out more broadly. And we should have done something similar for young boys and men. I don't know if that would have prevented the entire bulge of new infections among young people that we've seen in the '20s, but it surely would have brought it way down.

Dr. Zhang

OK, if I can summarize, here's what I've heard that we could have done better with respect to the social issues. We should have taken on the social issues much earlier than we did, which would have required recognition of the social and cultural complexities along with acceptance that society bears some of the responsibility for the epidemic. We should have implemented stronger policies to stop discrimination earlier than we did. We should have made better use of scientific data about the health effects of laws and social policies. And we needed to empower individuals through education and support systems, especially young people.

Anything else?

Mr. De Jong

I can tell you another thing that could have been done better. Religious groups and attitudes were such a huge problem. I wish they could have actually helped instead of hurting!

Dr. Zhang

Hey, come on, Joost. I asked everybody not to mention religion until we get to the third topic. I guess you just couldn't resist getting in a dig like that.

Dr. Bennett

I'd like to point out that I did better than Joost at following your instructions. I would have said that religious groups in the U.S. were often responsible for the lack of education about AIDS, HIV, and prevention. But you wanted us to wait, so I stopped myself from saying that.

Dr. Zhang

Thank you, Olivia. I appreciate your patience.

Anybody else have anything they want to add that isn't about money and isn't about religion?

Dr. Okafor

Yes, one more thing to point out. Different countries and regions dealt with the epidemic very differently. We certainly saw that in western Africa. Many west African countries were just slow to act. You'd think they would have learned from their friends in eastern and southern Africa. Or Russia, where there was such rapid growth in new HIV infections during the 2010s. They just ignored the problem. And there were similar problems in parts of Asia, the Middle East, North Africa, that also had growing numbers of new infections. I don't know the degree to which these differences were due to social issues, but I suspect a lot.

Dr. Bennett

I'm sure you're right. We also saw that in the U.S., for example, in the link between the opioid epidemic of the late 2010s and increases in HIV infection. We put off dealing with the opioid epidemic for far too long, and certainly part of the reason was social issues.

Dr. Zhang

Thank you.

Now I think it's time to move on to the next topic.

Did Religion Help or Hurt the Global AIDS Response?

Dr. Zhang

The final question I'd like you to answer is: did religion help or hurt the global AIDS response? Religion has been a controversial part of the AIDS story since the very beginning. And, frankly, it still is. Perhaps I'm naïve to hope for it, but it would be nice if this panel could come up with a definitive answer.

Rev. Morgan

May I start? I want to get a few words in here before Joost gets on his soap box again. I hope it is not controversial to say that faith-based institutions have been a vital part of providing services to people with HIV for a long time. We were on the front line from the very beginning. We were out there taking care of people long before there was any kind of treatment, and we're still out there. Studies over the entire fifty years of the epidemic have consistently shown that between twenty and forty percent of all HIV services are provided by faith-based institutions.

And the reason that we're providing these services is, first, that our faith compels us to help the sick, and second, that there are faith-based institutions everywhere. I remember a slide used

Rev. Emily Morgan:
I hope it is not controversial to say that faith-based institutions have been a vital part of providing services to people with HIV for a long time.

---

by Rick Warren of Saddleback Church in California, it must have been twenty-five years ago. It was a map of Rwanda that showed all of the medical facilities. There were just a few, kind of scattered around the country. And then he overlaid it with a map that showed all of the churches. A huge number, all over the place. His point was that faith communities have substantial organizational structures that they took advantage of in the AIDS epidemic. And still do.

And, in case you are wondering, HIV services are provided to anyone who is sick. We don't care how they got sick. We are just there to take care of them.

Dr. Zhang
What do you say, Joost? Is Emily right?

Mr. De Jong
Yes, of course she's right. Churches and other faith-based institutions were great at providing HIV services. That's not where the damage was done. The damage was all about the social issues that we just talked about. The stigma we talked about, it was largely driven by religion, by religious leaders who kept pushing these notions that AIDS was God's punishment for bad behavior.

Rev. Morgan
Wait a minute, that's a pretty old notion. You're living in the past, Joost. Yes, there was some of that in the beginning, but it didn't last long.

Mr. De Jong

Actually, it did last pretty long, a couple of decades at least. But even as it tapered off, those leaders kept emphasizing all of those so-called "bad" behaviors. That sure created a lot of stigma.

Imam Karume

We talk about stigma a lot as if it's just a single issue. It's much more complicated than that. Let me give you an example. I attended a meeting in Nairobi maybe twelve or fifteen years ago. It was structured as a dialogue between faith leaders and people living with HIV. And stigma came up a lot. But what struck me was the difference between stigma toward young people who have premarital sex and stigma toward men who have sex with men. It wasn't just degrees of difference. They were completely different attitudes. We were able to somehow tolerate premarital sex, but sex between men, in our culture, was just too abnormal for us to even think about it.

Dr. Bennett

In the U.S., we also had different kinds of stigma, but they worked out differently than in Africa. In the U.S., AIDS was initially seen as a gay disease, and to some degree that initial perception lasted for decades. So, if a woman became infected with HIV, there was always the question, "Wait a minute? How did she get it?" She got stigmatized.

Imam Karume

One other thing came out of that Nairobi meeting. We had both Christian and Muslim leaders, and our attitudes about stigma were really pretty similar. But we also had some data about levels of stigma in different parts of the country. The areas of Kenya that were predominantly Muslim had lower HIV prevalence than the predominantly Christian areas, but higher levels of stigma. And then, during the course of the next decade, we saw dramatic increases in new infections and prevalence in the Muslim-dominated sections.

[Editor's note: At this point, several demonstrators started shouting "RELIGION KILLS!" They continued for several minutes.]

Dr. Okafor
Can I interrupt here? Religion doesn't kill. It's the misuse of religion that kills. Look, and I'm talking to the demonstrators now, you've got to keep something in mind. One of the purposes of religion is to promote good behavior. There will be differences among different religions, like Christianity and Islam, and even within different branches of the same religion. But, in any case, it is still basically a moral code, guidance about how people ought to behave. And it's good to have guidelines like that. We want to be able to promote good behavior. We want to promote moral codes.

This leads to two very different issues. One issue is: what is the right moral code? A lot of the discussions and arguments about stigma and AIDS have been about what the right moral code is. But we're never going to get complete agreement on that. Arguments about the right moral code have been going on for millennia, and they'll keep going on for more millennia.

The second issue is: how do you promote a moral code without stigmatizing the people who don't follow it? Here is where I fault many religious groups and leaders. They can be too quick to judge and condemn. Instead, they could at least treat everybody with dignity and respect. Even if somebody's doing bad behavior according to your moral code, and even if they think your moral code is wrong, you can at least treat them with dignity and respect. Acknowledge the differences. But don't judge them so quickly. In my mind, that's where a lot of religious groups hurt the global AIDS response. If they hadn't been so quick to judge, then there would have been a lot less stigma, the key populations wouldn't have felt so marginalized, and we would have saved a lot more lives.

And for you demonstrators, you have to realize that you may not be able to change moral codes that people have believed for a long time. But you absolutely have the right to be treated with dignity and respect. You should demand that right, and we'll be there with you.

Imam Karume

You are reminding me of something the founder of INERELA+ always said, going back at least twenty-five years. That was Rev. Canon Gideon Byamugisha. He was an Anglican priest from Uganda, the first African religious leader to be open about being HIV-positive. He always said that, with respect to HIV and AIDS, we need to distinguish between two dimensions of human behavior. One is the moral dimension, like the moral codes you just talked about. Gideon used the phrase "lawful behavior," as in accordance with God's law. The other dimension of human behavior is safety—behavior that does or does not prevent HIV transmission. For this dimension, we look to our doctors and scientists for guidance. Gideon's point was that the two dimensions are different, but we religious people have a tendency to confuse or mix the two together. We needed to educate people about both dimensions.

Dr. Bennett

That's the point I wanted to make when we were discussing social issues. In the U.S., we were often unable to separate the moral and safe dimensions. That's why many of our schools didn't provide enough education about HIV and especially about methods of preventing HIV transmission.

Imam Ahmed Karume:
It was hard for religious leaders to deal with the social complexities of HIV and AIDS.

Rev. Morgan

You know, there were a lot of faith leaders and communities who actually did a pretty good job of educating, of treating people with dignity and respect, of providing counseling and support, of not judging, of not stigmatizing. They worked hard at it. They had specific programs aimed at eliminating stigma.

Imam Karume

Yes, I know. But not enough of them.

Rev. Morgan

Actually, it's really hard to know how many there were. We had lots of studies that showed the benefit of programs to reduce stigma in faith communities, but a lot of that was anecdotal. I do remember a study done maybe six or seven years ago. They identified some criteria for when a faith community is actively increasing stigma or actively decreasing stigma. Then they did surveys in several African countries, trying to come up with the percentage of the population that regularly worships at a faith community that increases stigma or decreases stigma. To use the words of the question to the panel: how many people were in faith communities that helped the AIDS response, and how many were in faith communities that hurt? To their surprise, they found that something like forty percent of the population worshipped at faith communities that hurt and less than ten percent at faith communities that helped. If we wanted to really make a dent in stigma, we needed those numbers swapped. We needed a lot more non-stigmatizers and a lot fewer stigmatizers.

Amb. Rogers

There's one other area where I think we needed more help from religion: global advocacy.

Rev. Morgan

How can you say that? Religious leaders have been global advocates for a long time! Canon Gideon was a strong advocate thirty or forty years ago. Or think back to the beginning of PEPFAR. Chris, you're at PEPFAR. You know the history. Religious advocacy played a big role in the creation of PEPFAR. President Bush started PEPFAR for moral reasons, not political ones, and many American religious leaders pushed him to do it. Also, many American evangelicals were strong advocates in the late 2000s. And then about twenty years ago, a group of religious leaders made a very strong statement at a meeting organized by UNAIDS. So it's not like religious leaders were quiet!

Dr. Okafor

I know. But somehow, that religious advocacy never quite made it to the forefront. Do you remember all the marches we used to have at previous AIDS conferences? It always struck me as odd and disappointing that there was barely any participation by religious leaders. There were never more than a few dozen. I'm glad to say that the demonstrations today in Durban included many more religious leaders. There were hundreds of them! And they were at the front of the marches. I just wish they had been that visible ten or twenty years ago.

Dr. Chibuzo Okafor:
Do you remember all the marches we used to have at previous AIDS conferences? It always struck me as odd and disappointing that there was barely any participation by religious leaders.

Amb. Rogers

And we didn't have that global advocacy during the critical period of time from 2015 to 2020. We really could have used some strong advocacy by prominent religious leaders. We needed them to be the global conscience, to make the case that ending AIDS was a moral imperative.

Dr. Zhang

Why do you think they didn't? Anybody have any thoughts on that?

Dr. Okafor

I don't know. I suspect part of it was complacency. Religious leaders thought AIDS was over, just like a lot of other people. Globally, there just wasn't a sense of urgency. It's not quite the same, but remember the Ebola outbreak in western Africa about fifteen years ago. The thing that really stopped it was when community leaders, especially religious leaders, got together and talked about what they needed to do. And they did it. And Christians and Muslims worked together to do it. And the reason they did it, and the reason they worked together, was that the situation was dire and urgent, and everybody could see that. Maybe back in that critical time period from 2015 to 2020, if prominent religious leaders had recognized the urgency and had gotten together to say something strong and loud, maybe that would have made a difference.

Imam Karume

I think another part of the reason was that it was hard for religious leaders to deal with the social complexities of HIV and AIDS. To fight Ebola, we needed to change some traditional practices, like funerals, for example. But the social complexities of HIV and AIDS are somehow harder to accept and harder to deal with. And that makes it harder to be strong advocates.

Dr. Bennett

And now, almost ten million people are dead, at least in part because religious leaders couldn't deal with the social complexities.

Dr. Zhang

Let me try to summarize this discussion so we can move on to questions from the audience. Remember, the question before us was: did religion help or hurt the AIDS response? I heard three answers. First, I think there was pretty broad consensus that religious organizations have done a really good job using their organizational structures to help with delivery of HIV services. Second, there were some, even many, religious leaders and communities who did quite well at helping to resolve the social issues, but there were probably not enough of them. On balance, more harm than help. And third, we sometimes had great global advocacy by religious leaders, but not when we needed it the most, in the late 2010s.

Anything else?

Rev. Morgan

Just to point out that we don't have the definitive answer you asked us for. Or rather, the definitive answer is both Yes and No. Religion definitely helped the global AIDS response in some ways, and it definitely hurt it in others. It will probably remain controversial for some time.

Dr. Zhang

I'm sure you're right.

Questions from the Audience

Dr. Zhang

Now I'd like to open it up to the audience. Please line up at the microphones in the aisles. It looks like you are doing that already. Now, you don't need to limit your questions to the three topics we focused on. Your questions can be about anything related to the AIDS epidemic.

Also, I should mention that we have made arrangements with the demonstration leaders to ensure that the demonstrators get to ask questions during this session. We've handed out about a half dozen little red cards to some of the demonstrators. As you stand in line, make sure you hold up your red card high so that we can see it from up here.

You first, at microphone number 3. It looks like you have a red card. Please start with your name and where you are from.

Question

My name is Mwenya Banda. My father, Paul Banda, was a Presbyterian minister in eastern Zambia. He was HIV-positive. He went public about his status in 2015, hoping to encourage others to seek testing and treatment. He was on ARVs, his viral load was suppressed, and he was leading a very productive life, providing spiritual help to hundreds of people. But in 2021, there began to be shortages of the medications. He started to take his medicine every other day, instead of every day, hoping to make it last. But he soon became ill. He died in 2025. My family and our community were devastated. My question to you is, why did my father die?

Imam Karume

I knew your father. I am so sorry that he died. We miss him. He was one of the best activists and advocates that we had, full of courage. We miss him. And he shouldn't have died. I know this isn't a good answer to your question, but your father was a victim of the lost political will that we talked about earlier on the panel. He was one of those eight to ten million people who shouldn't have died.

Dr. Zhang

Thank you. Next, microphone number 1. I see you also have a red card.

Question

My name is Oksana Silchenko. I come from Russia. I have been married to Andriy for six years. Andriy had been a drug addict before we got married, but I am proud to say that together we are now able to manage his addiction. We have recently learned that Andriy was infected by HIV during his addiction years, and now I am infected. My question to you is, why do I have HIV?

Mr. De Jong

First, I am glad that you and your husband were able to gain control over his addiction. Now, I know that you feel like life has treated you unfairly. And you're right. We've known for a long time, at least twenty years, that needle-exchange programs work to prevent HIV infection among people who inject drugs. But we were very slow to roll out those programs, especially in places that didn't recognize the reality and extent of drug use. If there had been a needle-exchange program in Russia, neither you nor your husband would have become infected with HIV. We failed you. I am sorry.

Dr. Zhang
Thank you. Next, microphone number 2.

Question
My name is Zendaya Moyo. I come from Harare. I'm sure you all remember the stockouts that happened in some places, when the supplies of medication ran out, especially in the first years of the 2020s. One of the effects of the stockouts was that many people lost trust in doctors and medical services. So then, when the first vaccine came out in 2024, nobody believed what the doctors said. That's why it took so long to roll out.

Rev. Morgan
Thanks for pointing that out. Yes, I remember. Many of the groups that we worked with were surprised at how much distrust there was and how it grew so quickly. I'm sure you're right about the effect that distrust had on the vaccine rollout.

Dr. Zhang
Thank you. Next, you over there at microphone number 3.

Question
My name is Patience Maduka. I come from a rural area in northern Malawi. Eight years ago, my cousin Vincent, the son of my father's sister, was born with HIV. Vincent died before his second birthday. My aunt, Vincent's mother, didn't go to a clinic during her

pregnancy. She knew that she might be HIV-positive, but she also knew that the clinic didn't have any more medication, so there was no point in going. My question to you is, why did my cousin die?

Dr. Thomas

I hate to say it, but the answer to your question is pretty easy. We've known how to prevent mother-to-child transmission for more than twenty years. All it took was to put that knowledge to good use. And, by the mid 2010s, we were well on track to ending MTCT. But then the cutbacks in the global response destroyed that progress. The world response failed your aunt and failed Victor.

Dr. Zhang

OK, now microphone number 2.

Question

My name is Mary Jefferson. I come from San Angelo, Texas, in the United States. My son Tyler was a star quarterback on his high school football team. Tyler was injured during his senior year and given opioids to relieve the pain. He became addicted and eventually joined a group of young addicts who shared their needles. Tyler became infected with HIV, but my health insurance wouldn't cover HIV treatment. Tyler died last year. Tell me, why did my son die?

Dr. Bennett

I'm very sorry to hear about your son. There is not a good answer to your question, because Tyler shouldn't have died. He was a victim of two challenges that we in the U.S. handled very badly. One was the opioid epidemic. We never should have let it grow as fast and as long it did. The other was needle-exchange programs. We knew they worked to prevent HIV transmission, but we were very slow to roll them out. Our country failed your son.

Dr. Zhang

OK. Microphone number 3, please.

Question

My name is Adila Ahmadi. I live in a village north of Mombasa, Kenya. I followed all the guidance that my Imam gave to us as girls. I was a virgin when I got married in 2022. Four years later my husband died from AIDS. He was a truck driver and must have become infected on one of his trips to southern Africa. After his death, I learned that I was HIV-positive. My question to you is, why do I have HIV?

Imam Karume

Thank you for sharing your story. I know it was difficult for you to do that. While your husband obviously has some responsibility for your infection, your religious leaders must also share the blame. You did everything right. We did not. We should have done a better job of educating and empowering both you and your husband. But we didn't. We just hoped that things would work out. I can only apologize and say that I wish we had done better.

Dr. Zhang

OK. Microphone number 2 again.

Question

My name is Ginny Mitchell. I come from the UK. There's one other interaction between religion and AIDS that's worth mentioning. I'm sure some of you remember Sally Smith. She was the UNAIDS special advisor for faith activities for about fifteen years in the 2000s and 2010s. She did a really interesting PhD thesis. She analyzed the wording of the various political declarations that had been made about AIDS over fifteen years at the UN, from 2000 through to 2016.

She showed that delegations from some countries that were closely aligned with certain religious traditions often pushed hard-line restrictive language. Strong and helpful religious voices got blocked out of the policy debate. The result was that the declarations and decisions mentioned the real needs of people most at risk of and impacted by HIV much less than many of us would have liked. I know that national programs got hampered as a result.

Dr. Nkosi
I'm glad you mentioned that. I remember Sally's thesis. It shed a whole new light on the way our international groups make decisions.

Dr. Zhang
Thank you. I'm looking for more red cards. Oh, yes, microphone number 4.

Question
My name is Rodrigo Mendoza. I live in Manila. I am a very active member of my church. In fact, my entire family is very devoted to the church and has been for many generations. Eight years ago, my son, Angelo, learned that he was HIV-positive. He and I talked about it and decided that he should seek advice from our church leaders. They rejected him. Angelo was devastated. Four days later, he committed suicide. My question to you is, why did my son die?

Dr. Okafor
I am very sorry to hear your story. This should never have happened. Unfortunately, religious institutions have always been slow to change. There were some significant initiatives in the mid 2010s that probably would have helped your son, but it has been very slow going. I wish we could have acted faster.

Dr. Zhang

Thank you. Now, microphone number 3.

Question

My name is Michael Robinson. I come from the United States, the state of Indiana. My husband Greg and I got married shortly after same-sex marriage became legal in the United States. He was HIV-positive. We were always careful, and I am still HIV-negative. In 2020, the policies changed in the United States, and he was no longer able to get health insurance. His health care costs went up quickly, and we couldn't afford his treatment. Greg died in 2026. My question to you is, why did Greg die?

Dr. Thomas

I am so sorry to hear this. Sadly, we in the U.S. were never really very good at dealing with health care. The big challenge for us was pre-existing conditions. We tried a bunch of different ways to ensure that health insurance was available for people with pre-existing conditions, which included HIV, but failed. Lately, I think we're finally finding more sensible ways to provide health care to everybody, including people with pre-existing conditions. But I'm sorry that it's too late for your husband.

Dr. Zhang

Thank you. I don't see any more red cards. Let's go to you on microphone number 2.

Question

My name is George Michalski. I come from San Francisco. As you look back, when do you think we hit the point of no return? If we had realized more quickly how bad the 2019 decision was, could we have recovered? Or by then, was it already too late?

Dr. Nkosi

Well, first, all of us on the panel hope, or really believe, that it still isn't too late, that somehow we can recover. But let me try to answer your question more directly. If we compare the actual expenditures with the original Fast Track targets for expenditures, there was a total shortfall of about ninety billion dollars over fifteen years. If we had tried to recover—starting say in 2023—in order to catch up, the annual investment would have had to be much higher than originally planned, partly to catch up and partly because of the extra new infections. The best estimate I've seen is that we would have had to increase the annual investment by fifteen or twenty billion dollars beginning in 2023. So, yes, it would have been possible to recover, but it would have cost a lot more overall than if we hadn't started cutting in the late 2010s.

You know, I just thought of this. We could tie these numbers to Charlize's comment. Our shortfall was about ninety billion dollars, and about eight or ten million people lost their lives needlessly. That means that the value of each of those lives is about ten thousand dollars. Is that what Charlize meant when she said we value some lives less than others? How many of us in this room like to think that we are worth a lot more than ten thousand dollars?

Dr. Zhang

Wow. That's a heavy thought! OK. I see one more red card. Microphone number 1.

Question

My name is Lindiwe Ndlovu. I live in Johannesburg. My daughter Thabise was born in 2008. When she was 14, Thabise hooked up with a Sugar Daddy who gave her financial security for a while. But, after six years, he left her. Thabise came home to live with me. We have recently learned that she is HIV-positive. We are fortunate that we have been able to get ARVs for her, but she is worried about her future. My question to you is, why does my daughter have HIV?

Amb. Rogers

Sadly, your daughter is still the picture of the AIDS epidemic. I remember in 2015 when we started the DREAMS program, we were specifically hoping to help young girls like your daughter. And the program actually worked pretty well, but it was eliminated as part of our funding cuts in 2021. I wish we had been able to keep it going and that we had been able to help your daughter. I am so sorry.

Dr. Zhang

Time for one more question. Microphone number 2.

Question

My name is Amanda Stevenson. I come from Chapel Hill, North Carolina, in the U.S. This whole discussion has been very intellectual, very clinical, which is what we would expect from a group of distinguished academics and scientists and doctors. I want to know how you feel. You can all see the signs around the edges of the auditorium, the ones that say "YOU LOST THE WAR AGAINST AIDS!" How do those signs make you feel?

Mr. De Jong

For me, it's angry. If I hadn't been on this stage, I would have been one of those people holding those signs. The world could have won the war, we knew what to do, but we didn't. We blew it! And now a whole lot of people are dead.

Amb. Rogers

I could use words like "sad" or "disappointed" or maybe even "guilty," but those words don't convey the real magnitude of my feelings. It's strange, I wasn't one of the people who made those fateful decisions ten or fifteen years ago, but I knew many of the decision makers. I keep asking myself, if I had just spent a little more time with them, if I had argued more, if I had been more articulate, would the decisions have gone the other way? I'm sure I could have done more. Maybe a little bit extra from me would have saved millions of lives. I don't know, but I hate to think I might have made the difference.

Dr. Nkosi

The thing that bothers me the most is that we always speak in large numbers, like fifty-three million people who have died, or forty-four million people living with HIV. Sometimes it seemed like we were just playing a big numbers game, how many billions of dollars are we going to spend, let's split the difference, what's my fair share. But the outcome of the game affected real people leading real lives. For them, it wasn't a game. They are the ones whose feelings really matter. And I feel awful for having been part of the game that left them dead or devastated.

Imam Karume

I can't speak for all religious leaders, but I think a lot of us feel ashamed that we didn't do enough. That's certainly how I feel. I remember something that a friend of mine once said. Rev. Phumzile Mabizela was the Executive Director of INERELA+ for many years. She once said to me, "If we can't do this…" She was speaking about people of faith dealing with the social issues like stigma. She said, "If we can't do this, what good are we?" Well, we couldn't do it. We could have done more, we should have done more. But we didn't. So now I ask, what good are we?

Dr. Zhang

Thank you, Joost, Chris, Munashe, Ahmed. I know it's hard to talk about our feelings, because we all know what could have been. For me, it's an overwhelming feeling of regret. We knew what to do, and we could easily have done it. But we didn't.

Closing Remarks

Dr. Zhang

Let me use that as a transition to the final part of this panel. What should we have done? Look again at the name of the panel, *How We Lost the War Against AIDS*. I'd like us to articulate the major mistakes that were made and the major opportunities that were missed. I don't want any rambling comments here. I want something specific, that if it had gone the other way, we might not have lost the war. Let's start with you, Ahmed, and then go down the line.

Imam Karume

I wish we had done a better job of educating our young people and of providing safe spaces and support for them during their formative years.

Dr. Nkosi

I really wish that the American government had provided stronger leadership during 2015 to 2020, not just at the medical and technical level, but at the global political level. They could have brought much more attention to the epidemic and to the urgency of persisting, of not throwing away all that we had gained.

Mr. De Jong

I wish that we had found ways that key populations could access prevention and treatment services without fear of discrimination or criminal persecution. Even when we couldn't eliminate laws, we should have been able to provide HIV services in a way that people didn't need to worry about getting arrested.

Rev. Morgan

I wish that more local religious communities had addressed stigma much earlier and much more strongly, and that we had had better data about what local religious communities were or were not doing.

Dr. Okafor

I wish that the countries in western Africa had recognized the challenges of HIV and AIDS much earlier, so that we could have prevented the bubble of infections among young people that occurred in the 2020s.

Dr. Bennett

I wish that we in the United States had been able to fully implement the national HIV program that was announced in 2019 with so much hope and promise.

Dr. Thomas

I wish that we had done a much better job of basing laws and policies on scientific evidence, going way back to the early days of the epidemic, focusing especially on preventing new infections.

Amb. Rogers

I wish that globally prominent religious leaders had spoken loudly, persistently, and in unison during the critical period in the late 2010s.

Dr. Zhang

Thank you.

To close this session, I'd like to quote Charlize Theron again. This is how she ended her speech in 2016:

> *Since the first International AIDS Conference in 1985, we have been counting up, all the way to 21. Now it's time for us to start counting down. We have set a goal to end the AIDS epidemic by 2030. There are seven more International AIDS Conferences between now and then. They must be our last.*

Obviously, we have failed to live up to her challenge. This isn't our last AIDS conference. But I hope we've learned enough in this session that we really can start counting down. And I dearly hope that we will never need another panel like this one.

Charlize Theron (2016)

The real reason we haven't beaten the epidemic boils down to one simple fact: We value some lives more than others. We value men more than women. Straight love more than gay love. White skin more than black skin. The rich more than the poor. Adults more than adolescents.

Dr. Munashe Nkosi (2030)

If someone had said in 2019 that our decision would kill eight to ten million of the "more valuable" lives, maybe we would have decided differently.

Panelists

Olivia Bennett, PhD

Dr. Bennett is the President and Chief Executive Officer of the Campaign to End AIDS in America, a leading AIDS advocacy organization in the United States. Dr. Bennett earned her PhD in Public Policy from the University of Chicago. In 2024, she was named to lead CEAA.

Joost De Jong

Mr. De Jong is the Executive Director of WHN, the Worldwide HIV Network. For many years, Mr. De Jong has been a prominent advocate for the human rights of people living with HIV or at risk of HIV infection. He was named the Executive Director of WHN in 2025.

Rafael González, MD

Dr. González is on the faculty of Universidade de São Paulo, where he leads the Medical School Public Hospital. He earned his undergraduate degree at Universidade Federal do Rio de Janeiro and completed his MD at the Universidade de São Paulo in 2009. In 2028, he was elected to serve a two-year term as President of the International AIDS Society. He is the Co-Chair of the 28th International AIDS Conference.

Ahmed Karume, BA

Imam Karume is the Executive Director of INERELA+, the International Network of Religious Leaders Living with or Personally Affected by HIV or AIDS. Imam Karume received his undergraduate degree at Umma University in Kenya and his religious training at the London Muslim Centre. He served numerous congregations in Kenya and then joined the staff of INERELA+ in 2023. He became Executive Director in 2028.

Emily Morgan, MTh, DD

Rev. Morgan is the Executive Director of Christian Health Alliance, an umbrella organization for a number of Christian non-governmental organizations. Rev. Morgan is an ordained pastor. She was educated at the Boston University School of Theology. She served as a health missionary in a variety of countries before joining CHA in 2021. She has been the Executive Director of CHA since 2028.

Munashe Nkosi, MD

Dr. Nkosi is the Executive Director of the Global Fund to Fight AIDS, Tuberculosis and Malaria. She received her medical degree from the University of Cape Town, specializing in Infectious Diseases. She joined WHO in 2006, serving in various positions before moving over to the Global Fund to become Executive Director in 2027.

Chibuzo Okafor, PhD

Dr. Okafor is the Director of African Projects for International Interfaith Relief Services. He earned his undergraduate degree in Health Sciences at the University of Lagos and a PhD in Public Health from the University of Nigeria. He has served with IIRS for more than twenty years at many locations around the world. He was named Director of Africa Projects in 2027 and is based in Lagos.

Christopher Rogers, MD, PhD

Amb. Rogers is the United States Global AIDS Coordinator. He directs the PEPFAR program for the United States Government. He earned his PhD in International Development from Stanford University. He worked for many years at USAID before returning to Harvard Medical School, where he earned an MD with a specialty in Epidemiology. He joined PEPFAR in 2016 and was selected to lead the agency in 2023.

Jaylen Thomas, MD, PhD

Dr. Thomas is the Director of the Centers for Disease Control and Prevention in the United States. He earned an MD in Primary Care from Columbia University and then a PhD in Public Health from Johns Hopkins University. He served for many years at UNAIDS and WHO before being named the Director of the CDC in 2022.

Zhang Xiu Ying, PhD

Dr. Zhang is the Director-General of the World Health Organiza-tion. She earned her undergraduate degree at Tsinghua University and her PhD from the University of Oxford, with a specialization in International Health Policy. During her twenty-year career, she has worked for numerous international health organizations. She was selected to lead the Global Fund to Fight AIDS, Tuberculosis and Malaria in 2026.

"How We Lost the War Against AIDS"
Recorded by SA Media Consultants
Durban, South Africa
29 July 2030

Afterword

I hope this is a work of fiction, but it might not be. The AIDS epidemic is at a tipping point. If we tip in the wrong direction, we will have a future like the one depicted in this transcript of a future panel at a future AIDS conference. Fortunately, a tragic future is not inevitable. If we collectively do what we know how to do, we will have a future like the one depicted in the other half of this book, a transcript from a future panel titled *How We Won the War Against AIDS*.

David R. Barstow

June 2019

Corvallis, Oregon, USA

How We WON the War Against AIDS

Transcript of a Plenary Session
28th International AIDS Conference
Durban, South Africa
29 July 2030

Note from the Editor

There was an unusually large amount of media coverage of the 2030 International AIDS Conference, recently held in Durban, South Africa. Much of the media coverage was related to one specific panel session and the massive demonstrations that occurred outside the conference center while the panel was being held. Given this heightened interest, members of the Program Committee of the IAC have decided to make publicly available a complete transcript of the panel session. The transcript has been compiled from video recordings of the panel session. The words are those spoken by the panelists and audience members, except for minor edits to improve the flow.

David R. Barstow, Editor
5 August 2030
Corvallis, Oregon, USA

Question from the Audience
You're sitting up on a stage with a big sign that says, "HOW WE WON THE WAR AGAINST AIDS." How does that make you feel?

Mr. De Jong
For me, it's joy, of course, but also sadness. I'm sure we could have won the war quicker and better, and then some of the people who died might still be here with us.

Amb. Rogers
I remember back in the late 2010s, we could so easily have given up, or even just slowed down. And then we'd be here on a stage with a sign that says, "HOW WE LOST THE WAR AGAINST AIDS." I can't imagine how depressing that would have been.

Dr. Nkosi
I keep thinking about the millions of people whose lives were saved. Every one of those people is a living, breathing, human being, with family and friends and hopes and dreams. They are the ones whose feelings really matter.

Imam Karume
I know that pride is a dangerous sin, but in all honesty, I have to admit to feeling a little pride that we religious folk were so instrumental in coping with the social issues.

Introduction

Dr. González

Could you all please find seats so we can get started. I know there was a lot of commotion and confusion outside the hall, and that has delayed the start of the session. You can all help us get going if you take your seats.

While you are taking your seats, I'd like to update you on the demonstrations that took place throughout Durban today. We believe they are the largest demonstrations in the history of the AIDS epidemic. The police have estimated that over 50,000 people participated. I know that we all have seen demonstrations at previous AIDS conferences. This is perhaps the first time that the demonstrations have had such a celebratory tone.

For we do indeed have something to celebrate. As indicated by the title of the panel, *How We Won the War Against AIDS*, we are celebrating success in one of the greatest humanitarian initiatives in history.

[Editor's note: At this point, there was prolonged applause, lasting several minutes.]

It's amazing to be able to celebrate like this!

OK, it looks like things have settled down in the auditorium. Let's get started.

My name is Dr. Rafael González. It has been an honor to serve as the President of the International AIDS Society for the past two years. In that position, I am one of the Co-Chairs of this conference, the 28th International AIDS Conference.

This is now the third time that the International AIDS Conference has been held in Durban. Each time has marked a significant turning point in the AIDS epidemic.

The 13th IAC was held here in July 2000. It was the first time that the AIDS conference had been held in Africa and marked the global recognition of the magnitude of the AIDS epidemic.

Sixteen years later, the 21st IAC was held here in July 2016. It marked the first time that we believed we might actually be able to end AIDS. We had achieved remarkable progress, really amazing progress, in getting people with HIV on ARV treatment. And there was a strong sense that we had it in our power to end AIDS as a public health threat by 2030.

Now it is 2030, and we are here in Durban to mark our success. We have used the power we had, and we can now say that we have eliminated HIV and AIDS as public health threats.

[Editor's note: The audience broke into spontaneous applause that lasted several minutes.]

Now, in the final session of this conference, we have assembled a special panel, partly to help us celebrate our success, our victory over AIDS, and partly to look back to find lessons that will be helpful when we face future epidemics. How did we win the war against AIDS?

The panel will be moderated by Dr. Zhang Xiu Ying, the Director-General of the World Health Organization. Dr. Zhang, could you please introduce the other panelists and start the discussion.

Dr. Zhang

Thank you, Dr. González.

So the question is: how did we win the war against AIDS? We have invited eight panelists with distinguished backgrounds to help us answer this question. On the stage here with me, from your left to your right, we have:

Imam Ahmed Karume, the Executive Director of INERELA+, the International Network of Religious Leaders Living with or Personally Affected by HIV or AIDS.

Dr. Munashe Nkosi, the Executive Director of the Global Fund to Fight AIDS, Tuberculosis and Malaria.

Mr. Joost De Jong, the Executive Director of WHN, the World-wide HIV Network, an advocacy group for people living with HIV.

Rev. Emily Morgan, the Executive Director of Christian Health Alliance, a consortium of Christian NGOs.

Dr. Chibuzo Okafor, the Director of African Projects for International Interfaith Relief Services, a coalition of relief service organizations from a variety of religious traditions.

Dr. Olivia Bennett, on the faculty of Yale University in the School of Public Health. She was the President and Chief Executive Officer of the Campaign to End AIDS in America from 2024 through the closing of the organization in 2027.

Dr. Jaylen Thomas, the Director of the Centers for Disease Control and Prevention in the United States.

Amb. Christopher Rogers, who served as the United States Global AIDS Coordinator from 2023 to 2028. He ran PEPFAR during the last five years of its existence.

You can find more information about our panelists in your printed program.

I should add that the panelists today will be speaking as individuals, not as representatives of the organizations they work for. Opinions they express do not necessarily represent official positions of their organizations.

You may notice that the panelists are primarily public health experts, AIDS activists, and religious leaders. We have several scientists and doctors, but their careers have not focused on research or providing medical services directly to patients. That was a deliberate choice when we planned this panel. We won't be discussing the science of HIV and AIDS. That's not to undervalue the remarkable scientific and medical achievements. Without them, there would have been no hope of winning. But the hardest part of winning the war against AIDS has been the difficulty of using the knowledge effectively.

I will start this session by reviewing the basic epidemiological data from the fifty-year history of the AIDS epidemic. Then we will have open discussion among the panelists about three specific topics: funding, social drivers, and religion. In order to stimulate a livelier discussion, I have asked the panelists not to discuss the topics amongst themselves prior to their appearance on this panel. Of course, knowing the panelists as I do, it seems quite likely that they ignored my request!

Following the discussions about the three topics, we will open the panel to questions from the floor. We hope to have about twenty minutes for questions. We will then have brief closing statements by the panelists.

Let's get started.

Fifty Years of the AIDS Epidemic

Dr. Zhang

You have all seen this chart [*Figure 1, below*] before. It shows the annual rates of new HIV infections and AIDS-related deaths in the fifty years since the epidemic began in 1980. This is worldwide.

To quickly review the data, there was a rapid increase of new infections during the first fifteen years, peaking at 3.4 million in 1995, after which the rate of new infections began to decline. The decline has been pretty steady, except for a few years at the end of the 2010s. We project that the number of new infections in 2030

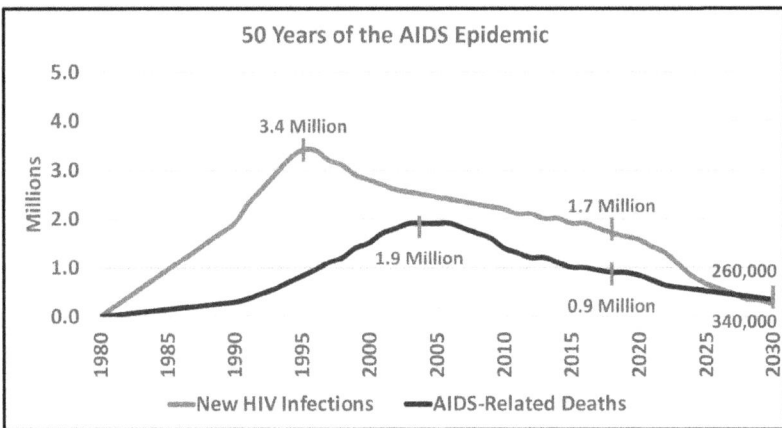

Figure 1—Fifty Years of the AIDS Epidemic

will be about 260,000 and will continue to decline in the foreseeable future.

The annual number of deaths from AIDS-related causes rose rapidly through the mid 2000s, at which point it also began to decline. Progress in reducing deaths has been pretty steady since its peak, with the exception of the same few years at the end of the 2010s. We project that there will be about 340,000 AIDS-related deaths in 2030. These also will continue to decline in future years.

During the fifty years of the epidemic, a total of about forty-four million people have died. Several years ago, we were worried that the number of deaths might ultimately go above sixty or seventy million, which would have been more than the number of people who died during World War II, the deadliest military war that the world has ever experienced. Fortunately, we were short of that, although still ahead of the death count for every other military war. So the war against AIDS still qualifies as one of the deadliest wars in human history.

Now, in looking at this chart, there are several time periods of particular interest. Certainly, the most important is right now, where we can see that we have brought HIV and AIDS under control. That's why we can have this panel with such a remarkable title, *How We Won the War Against AIDS*!

[Editor's note: The audience broke into spontaneous applause that lasted several minutes.]

But looking backward, we can also see the two peaks, the peak for new HIV infections in the mid 1990s and the peak of AIDS-related deaths in the mid 2000s. The first was when intensive prevention programs in sub-Saharan Africa began to have an effect. The second was when ARV treatment programs became more widespread, thanks largely to PEPFAR and the Global Fund.

One other interesting period, a little less obvious, was near the end of the 2010s, when there was a slowdown in progress for a few years. The slowdown in progress is also apparent in this chart [*Figure 2, below*] that shows treatment coverage for the twenty-year period between 2010 and 2030.

As seen on this chart, the number of people living with HIV has grown steadily from thirty-two million to about forty-two million. The number of people who know their status has gone up a little faster, and pretty steadily, except for a slight slowdown at the end of the 2010s. The number on treatment rose quickly from 2010 through 2018 but then slowed for a few years before rising again. The number of people who achieved viral suppression also rose steadily, from five million in 2010 to almost thirty-eight million now. Again, there was that little two-year slowdown at the end of the 2010s.

Most of you recall the Fast Track program, initiated by UNAIDS in 2015 with the goal of quickly gaining control of the epidemic by 2020 and then eliminating HIV and AIDS as public health threats by 2030. This was part of that optimistic mood of the 2016 Durban conference. The intermediate goal for 2020 was described as 90-90-90:

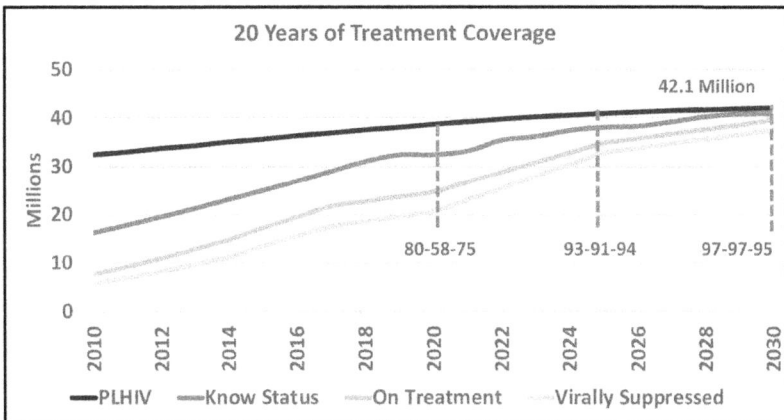

Figure 2—Twenty Years of Treatment Coverage

90% of people living with HIV know their status, 90% of them are on treatment, and 90% of them have reached viral suppression. We actually didn't achieve 90-90-90 until 2025. In 2020, we were only at 84-76-84. In 2025, we reached 93-91-94. We are currently at 97-97-95, which means that almost 90% of people living with HIV have achieved viral suppression.

Here's one more chart [*Figure 3, below*].

As you know, the ratio of incidence to prevalence has been used for the past decade as a single indicator of epidemic control. A ratio below 0.030 is generally thought to represent control of the epidemic. We were on a steady trajectory downward, with a hope of reaching the threshold about ten years ago. But then we had that same slowdown in the late 2010s before moving downward again. We crossed the 0.030 threshold in 2023 and, in fact, have continued the downward trend. We are now at 0.006.

Any comments before we go on to the three topics?

Dr. Okafor

Just one. You've already pointed out the slowdowns in the curves in the late 2010s. That happened right about the time that we were

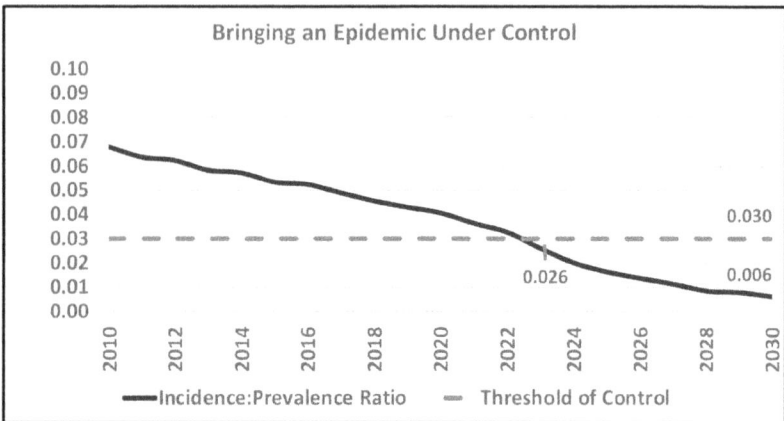

Figure 3—Bringing an Epidemic Under Control

worried that the rate of new infections might go up, especially among young people. That was a big worry in my home country of Nigeria. It was certainly a relief when we saw that our worst fears weren't going to happen.

Dr. Zhang
Yes, you're right. I'm sure all of us felt that sense of relief when the infection rates started to go down again.

Dr. Thomas
And a major factor in that was PrEP, pre-exposure prophylaxis. Remember, it got off to a slow start in the late 2010s, but then it grew to widespread use in the early 2020s. That was certainly one big factor in reducing new infections.

Also, remember our first vaccine? It came out in 2024. The vaccine was only 60% effective, but it was still a significant help to people who used it. The rollout was a little slower than we had hoped, but it began to have a significant epidemiological effect a few years ago. Our best estimate is that the current rate of new HIV infections is about 10% less than it would have been without the vaccine.

Dr. Zhang
Yes, I believe you are right.

OK, now let's start on our first topic.

Why Did Funding for AIDS Fluctuate?

Dr. Zhang

The first topic is money. This chart *[Figure 4, below]* shows the overall global investment in the AIDS response for the past twenty years.

Now this is global investment—the total amount of money spent on the AIDS response worldwide: PEPFAR, Global Fund, internal domestic sources, rich countries, poor countries, NGOs, everything. As you can see, it was at $15 billion in 2010, rose for a few years, peaking at about $21.5 billion, then took a small drop,

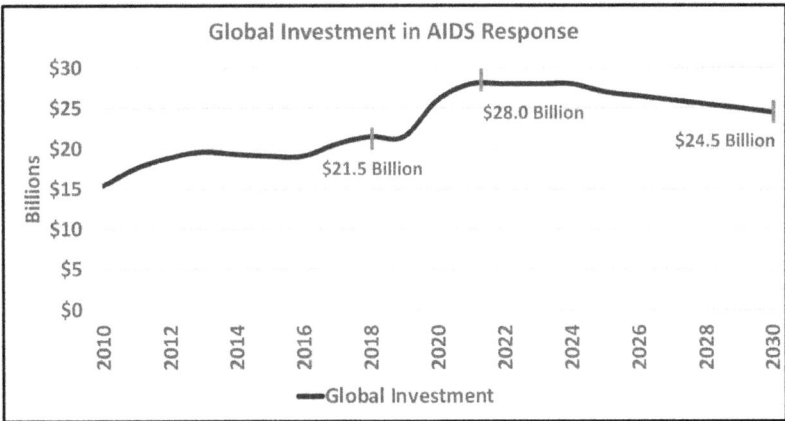

Figure 4—Global Investment in AIDS Response

Dr. Zhang Xiu Ying:
Fifteen years ago, who would have guessed that we'd reach a time when PEPFAR would no longer be needed?

---

then an even bigger leap, held steady at $28 billion for several years, and gradually declined to about $25 billion in 2030.

Dr. Nkosi

Before we go any further, let's remind ourselves of something that isn't on this chart, namely the early 2000s. That's when the global AIDS effort really started to take off. I was a junior member of the South African delegation to the special session of the UN General Assembly in 2001. That's when Peter Piot made his famous comment about "two possible futures." That's when the Declaration of Commitment on HIV/AIDS was agreed to. Then came the Global Fund, followed by PEPFAR. If we want to know how we won the war against AIDS, we certainly have to highlight the start of what would become one of the greatest global humanitarian efforts of modern times, perhaps of all time.

Dr. Zhang

Yes, you are certainly right. That special session of the UN marked a turning point. And without the Global Fund and PEPFAR, who knows where we would be right now? That was so long ago, more than a quarter century, that it has become simply an assumed part of the global response. Thank you for the reminder.

Amb. Rogers

And, of course, PEPFAR is no longer here. I have to say that it is a delight to see this investment chart, especially what happened in the past few years. Remember, the reason that PEPFAR was closed in 2028 was that it was no longer needed. The high-burden countries no longer needed funding from PEPFAR. The fact that PEPFAR ended doesn't even register at all on the global investment trends.

Dr. Zhang

Right. Fifteen years ago, who would have guessed that we'd reach a time when PEPFAR would no longer be needed?

Now back to this chart. There's a correlation with the previous charts. The fluctuations in funding in the late 2010s were at about the same time as the slowdowns in the epidemiological charts. Presumably, there was a cause and effect here: the slowdown in global investment contributed to the slowing down of progress against HIV and AIDS.

The deeper questions are: (1) why did investment slow down in the late 2010s? And (2) why did investment go up so dramatically in 2020?

Let's look at the first question first. Why did investment drop in the late 2010s? What do you think?

Dr. Okafor

Well, for one thing, the slowdown wasn't really a surprise. The global political will had been weakening for several years. The 2016 UN High-Level Meeting on AIDS was a difficult meeting, with lots of arguing about the right amount of funding. The UNAIDS Fast Track program wanted more aggressive funding than many countries were prepared to commit to. And then, at the 2016 Global

Fund replenishment meeting a few months later, it was hard to even get what we got. So the warning signs were there.

Dr. Thomas

I think a lot of the lost political will was AIDS fatigue. Governments were simply tired of thinking about AIDS. I know that was the case in the U.S. And think about the Sustainable Development Goals. AIDS had been a big piece of the Millennium Development Goals fifteen years earlier, but it got less attention with the SDGs in 2015. AIDS fatigue was certainly one cause of the weakened political will.

Amb. Rogers

Another big part of it was complacency. Many, many people thought that the AIDS crisis was over. Why did we need to pour in more money? Other issues became more prominent, like climate change, mass migrations, economic inequality. And then there were other diseases, like Ebola. AIDS had been a top-level issue in the 2000s, but by the end of the 2010s, AIDS was much less visible, and governments spent less time and energy on it.

Mr. De Jong

I think it was more indifference, rather than complacency. Complacency is when you think things are OK. Indifference is when you don't really care whether or not they are OK. And, sometimes I think it was even hostility, anger that so much money had been spent on other people and other countries. The countries should have been able to take care of themselves. Remember, the populist and nationalist movements in the U.S. and Europe peaked in the late 2010s, and those movements always had an element of anger and resentment toward other people and other countries and other problems.

Rev. Morgan

Remember, the AIDS crisis was largely seen as rich countries providing all the money and poor countries spending it, so the anger and resentment were understandable. Of course, the real funding picture wasn't that simple, and over time the high-burden countries gradually took over more and more of the financial cost. But what do you think would have happened if that transition had happened sooner? If the high-burden countries had covered more of the costs earlier, and if they had used those funds more effectively, then maybe there wouldn't have been that slowdown at the end of the 2010s.

Dr. Zhang

Well, as Chris has already pointed out, the transition did ultimately happen, which was why PEPFAR was closed down two years ago.

Now let's go on to the second question. Why did investment go up so dramatically in 2020? And for this question, I think we can very usefully focus on a single event, namely the Global Fund replenishment in 2019. The Global Fund had made its investment case for an increase of about 15%. There was a lot of nervousness in the months prior to the meeting in Lyon, a real fear that funds would be cut. But, and this was probably the real surprise in the funding story, the Global Fund partners agreed to the 15% increase. And that decision triggered other funding decisions. Like the recipient countries. As I recall, they raised their domestic funding for AIDS by almost 50%. That was hugely important! In terms of dollars, the increase in domestic funding was more important than the Global Fund decision that triggered it. That's what we saw on that chart. The 2019 replenishment decision was the key that started the ball rolling. Why did it go the way it did?

Dr. Zhang Xiu Ying:
The key event was the Global Fund replenishment decision in 2019. Thanks in part to American leadership, the Global Fund was increased instead of decreased. If that decision had gone the other way, we wouldn't be here talking about winning the war against AIDS.

Dr. Nkosi

Yes, it was a surprise, but I think the reason is pretty simple: American leadership. For whatever reason, the Americans decided to push very hard for the increase and committed the funds for their share. And they did it publicly. It became a major goal for the American government, and they pushed very hard. A lot of us were surprised, because for a couple of years, all we had seen were signs of weakening American leadership. Something changed, and that's what led to the 2019 replenishment decision.

Imam Karume

You're giving an awful lot of credit to the Americans. A lot of other countries also pushed for the replenishment increase. Like France. They hosted the meeting, and they came out early on pushing for the increase.

Dr. Nkosi

Yes, I know that, but in the context of that time, it had to be the Americans. If they hadn't pushed so hard, I really don't think it would have happened. They were the ones who had to reassert leadership and reinvigorate the global political will that had gotten so weak.

Dr. Zhang

OK, let's assume it was the Americans. Why do you think the Americans chose to take the lead? As Munashe has said, a lot of us were surprised. Quite happily, but none the less surprised.

Amb. Rogers

Well, I was there, of course. I saw it happen, and I still don't know why. The divisions in American politics back then were pretty strong. But PEPFAR and the Global Fund had always had good bipartisan support. Perhaps everybody saw it as a way to get something done together. Or perhaps it was the perception that cutting back would amount to defeat, throwing away all the great progress that had been made. And I suppose there were other things. In any case, I'm sure we are all very glad that it happened.

Dr. Thomas

That was also the time that the U.S. made a sudden big push on domestic HIV policy. U.S. domestic policy had been kind of dormant for several years, but then there was a burst of energy in 2019. I suspect that the actions on both the domestic front and on the international front were somehow related. You may remember that President Trump briefly mentioned HIV and AIDS in his State of the Union address in early 2019. He talked mostly about domestic policy, but, and I remember the words very clearly, he said, "and beyond." That was beyond the U.S. borders.

Dr. Bennett

I'm pretty sure the two were related. Most of the discussions in the U.S. in early 2019 were about the domestic strategy, including allocation of some new funds for the *Ending the HIV Epidemic* program that was focused on certain regions and populations, as well as Medicaid expansion in many states that had not previously expanded it. And then, only a few months later, the discussions broadened to include the global epidemic and the need for the United States to continue its strong leadership role. The timing couldn't have been purely coincidental.

Dr. Nkosi

Well, in any case, whatever led to it, we are all certainly grateful for the American leadership and for the 2019 Global Fund decision. I've seen some analyses of what would have happened if the replenishment decision had gone the other way, if the Global Fund had been reduced instead of increased. It depends on the magnitude of the reduction, of course, but the estimates are generally that between eight and ten million lives would have been lost if the Global Fund had been cut. So that Global Fund decision in 2019 saved many millions of lives.

Dr. Zhang

Thank you all. Let me see if I can summarize what you have said. The funding slowdown in the late 2010s was the result of several factors—AIDS fatigue, complacency, or indifference—but it mostly came down to a loss of political will. Fortunately, that didn't last long, and the key event was the Global Fund replenishment decision in 2019. Thanks in part to American leadership, the Global Fund was increased instead of decreased. If that decision had gone the other way, we wouldn't be here talking about winning the war against AIDS.

With that, I'd like to move on to our next topic.

How Did We Address
the Social Issues?

Dr. Zhang

The next topic is about everything except money. Other than the slowdown at the end of the 2010s, there was, generally speaking, enough money. But the AIDS epidemic isn't only about money. It has been complicated and exacerbated by a variety of social issues. Since the epidemic is now under control, we must have addressed these social issues well enough. How did we do that?

Amb. Rogers

Do you remember what Jonathan Mann said? Some of you may be too young to remember him. About forty years ago, he was the leader of the first WHO AIDS initiative, and something of a visionary, putting a lot of effort into human rights. I don't remember exactly what he said, but it went something like this:

> *AIDS is a social problem…*
> *…with some medical aspects.*

In other words, in many ways, the social drivers were more important than medical issues. But, especially during the first few decades of the epidemic, we spent a lot more money on science and medicine than we spent to address the social drivers. If Jonathan Mann was right, then we were spending all our money on the least important aspects. The medical and scientific work obviously produced amazing results, so it was certainly worth the money that was spent. But we should have paid a lot more attention to the social issues a lot earlier.

Dr. Nkosi

Yes, you're right. And I'll bet it would have even been cheaper in the long run. If we had done a better job with the social drivers earlier, then we might not even have needed the 2019 increase in the Global Fund.

Dr. Zhang

Let me add that we had this distinction in mind when we planned this panel. As I mentioned earlier, we won't be discussing the medical aspects of the epidemic. Figuring out how to deal with the social drivers was in many ways much more complicated.

Amb. Rogers

You know, there are some social drivers that apply to all epidemics, things like malnutrition, unsanitary water, poverty, mobile populations, incarceration, weak medical delivery systems. In this conversation, let's focus on the social drivers that are specific to HIV and AIDS. Most of these social drivers are related to the modes of transmission. For example, in addition to women's biological vulnerability, they are also vulnerable to HIV infection through sexual activity when they have a lower social status than men.

Mr. De Jong

There's also stigma, of course. Many people associate HIV with activities that they consider bad. Things like sex outside of marriage, same-sex relationships, injection drug use, transgender people, sex work. All of those are considered bad in one way or another by large segments of the population in many societies.

[Editor's note: At this point, several demonstrators rose from their seats and started walking around silently carrying signs that said, "STIGMA KILLS."]

Dr. Zhang *[addressing the demonstrators]*

Please take your seats. Remember, we are on your side. We know that stigma has killed a lot of people in the AIDS epidemic. And we know that stigma will persist and that we will have to keep fighting it. But we're also glad that we've made so much progress against it.

Joost, could you finish your thought, please?

Mr. De Jong

Well, it's not very complicated. When behavior is considered "bad," it leads to judgmental attitudes, which lead to stigma and social isolation. And these, in turn, cause people to avoid testing and treatment.

Dr. Bennett

We certainly saw those effects of stigma in the United States. For example, black gay men were doubly stigmatized, and their rates of HIV infection were astronomical. At one point, we feared that the HIV prevalence rate would reach 50%. Fortunately, the U.S. domestic plan included programs specifically focused on working with gay black men, and they were quite successful.

Dr. Thomas

You know, we have lots of studies about the effect of stigma on the AIDS epidemic. So we know that the effects of stigma are real. The data show that fear of rejection by society often stops people from seeking testing and treatment, even when they think they may have HIV. And then there's self-worth. Stigma decreases a person's sense of self-worth, which leads to poor health decisions, not only about testing and treatment, but also about prevention.

Dr. Nkosi

And don't forget outright discrimination, discriminatory behavior. We saw a lot of discrimination in health clinics, churches, places of work. Many people were actually fired from work for being HIV-positive, even though it had nothing to do with their job. We had discrimination all over the place. And discrimination just reinforces stigma and the low sense of self-worth.

Mr. De Jong

And criminalization. Many places had laws against behavior that was seen as anti-social or against the norm. And obviously, fear of criminal prosecution stopped a lot of people from getting tested for HIV and from accessing prevention services. You're not going to seek help if you think you're going to get arrested!

Dr. Thomas

Do you remember the effect of travel restrictions? People unable to travel to the U.S and other countries, or who interrupted their treatment to be able to travel. You can imagine how dangerous that was.

Rev. Morgan

Basically, what we're saying here is that, for a variety of reasons, there were several population groups that were at increased risk of HIV infection. And the thing about them was that almost all of the key populations were somehow outside of mainstream society; they were marginalized. And the very fact that they were marginalized was part of the problem. As we know, HIV thrives among the marginalized.

Dr. Nkosi

Don't forget, some of the vulnerable populations were part of mainstream society, like young girls and women. Of course, they were often marginalized after the fact if they became infected by HIV.

Dr. Zhang

Yes, vulnerable and at-risk populations were marginalized. And, in many places, they still are. But somehow, in the context of the AIDS epidemic, we dealt successfully with marginalization, stigma, discrimination. What was it that we did?

Imam Karume

Well, it took a long time, but eventually we began to recognize and accept that society had some responsibility in the spreading AIDS epidemic. For the first several decades, the emphasis was always on individual personal responsibility for prevention. Remember the ABC strategy first rolled out in Uganda in the late 1990s? For those who don't know about this, the ABC stood for "Abstain, Be faithful, use a Condom." That is totally focused on the individual, as if society doesn't share any of the responsibility. Of course, personal responsibility is very important, but it's not everything. What about poverty that forces young girls to choose between two bad alternatives? Or laws that push some groups of people into hiding, where diseases like HIV can thrive? Or widespread gender-based violence, where it isn't even possible to take personal responsibility?

Mr. De Jong

You know, emphasizing personal responsibility actually increases stigma. Think about ABC, what it's really saying. "Abstaining from sex is the best thing to do, but if you can't abstain, at least be faithful to your spouse, and if you can't even do that, then use a condom when you're being unfaithful." Condoms are the third best option. If you use a condom, it's because you can't succeed at the two best options. What a failure you are!

Dr. Bennett

In the U.S., this notion of personal responsibility came up in our debates about health insurance. We always had trouble dealing with pre-existing conditions, and I think that some of our difficulty was an unconscious belief that any pre-existing condition was somehow the person's fault. And, of course, infection with HIV was seen as a prime example of a pre-existing condition that resulted from irresponsible personal behavior. But, at least in the case of HIV, we were able to get past that perception when we launched the domestic strategy in 2019.

Imam Karume

And the good news is that we eventually realized there was also societal responsibility. And if we were going to end the AIDS epidemic, then we had to accept that responsibility and do something about it. As I look back, it seems to me that the 2010s were the decade when we really began to accept societal responsibility. We found a good balance between personal and societal responsibility.

Dr. Zhang
OK, but what was it that we did?

Amb. Rogers
Well, for one thing, we accepted the reality that there were key populations that were at increased risk, and we started rolling out programs that were specifically focused on those populations. For example, needle-exchange programs for people who inject drugs. So, we ended up with lots of different programs, for people facing domestic violence, for sex workers and their clients, for people in prison. We were very focused on the places and populations where the epidemic, and the risks, were highest.

Dr. Bennett
That was a central point of the U.S. domestic HIV and AIDS strategy throughout the 2020s. It included many programs specifically focused on the needs of key and vulnerable populations.

Mr. Okafor
Also, we gradually implemented laws and policies that stopped discrimination. It took a while for them to have their full effect, but that was a very important part of it. And just as important, we dealt with the underlying paradigms that drive stigma.

Mr. De Jong
And, of course, we had to deal with criminalization. Laws against same-sex behavior were the most obvious, but there were others, like travel restrictions. We were successful in repealing many of these laws. And when we were not able to repeal the laws, we found

Rev. Emily Morgan:
PEPFAR started the DREAMS program in the late 2010s. It did a really good job of helping young girls. And then PEPFAR launched a similar program for young boys in 2021 called HOPES. I am certain that these programs were key to preventing the bulge of new infections among young people that we feared we would see in the '20s.

---

ways for people to get HIV services, both prevention and treatment, without fearing arrest and criminal prosecution. Sometimes it was formal sanctuary zones, sometimes it was informal agreements between service providers and police. So it was different in different places, but in most places, we eventually figured out something that worked.

Imam Karume

You know, another area where we did pretty well was empowering people to take care of themselves. It took a while, of course, but eventually we developed widespread education programs, both about the nature of HIV and AIDS and about the various options for preventing HIV transmission.

Rev. Morgan

And we developed strong support systems for individuals, both those with HIV and those at risk of infection. This was really important for young people. PEPFAR started the DREAMS program in the late 2010s. It did a really good job of helping young girls. And, thanks to growth in funding, PEPFAR was able to roll it out more broadly. And then PEPFAR launched a similar program for young boys in 2021 called HOPES. I am certain that these programs were key to preventing the bulge of new infections among young people that we feared we would see in the '20s.

Mr. De Jong

I'd like to mention one more thing: messaging campaigns about viral suppression. It seems like a little thing, but do you remember the "U=U" campaign? "Undetectable Equals Untransmittable." It had an interesting side effect that I don't know that we anticipated. It put a real dent in self-stigma. It gave people living with HIV a certain sense of dignity. Somehow, it helped them realize that they were normal people, that they could rejoin the human race.

[Editor's note: At this point, there was applause from the crowd for several minutes.]

Dr. Zhang

Joost, thanks for mentioning that. I had forgotten about that campaign.

OK. We have a list of some of the important things we did: programs focused on key populations, laws and policies against discrimination, ways of dealing with criminalization, addressing stigma, education and empowerment, especially of young people, and campaigns to help PLHIV recover their dignity. That's actually a pretty good list.

Now, why did we do all of these things? What motivated us?

Mr. De Jong

I never thought I'd say this, but I think religious leaders and communities had a lot to do with it.

Amb. Christopher Rogers:
People gradually began to realize that the boundaries between the marginalized and the rest of society are not impervious.

Dr. Zhang

Hey, Joost, remember I asked you not to mention religion until we get to the third topic.

Dr. Bennett

I'd like to point out that I did better than Joost at following your instructions. I would have said that religious groups in the U.S. were instrumental in changing the way our children learned about AIDS, HIV, and prevention. But you wanted us to wait, so I stopped myself from saying that.

Dr. Zhang

Thank you, Olivia. I appreciate your patience.

Mr. De Jong

You know, it may not be possible to separate religion from these social issues.

Dr. Zhang

Let's give it a try.

Amb. Rogers

Well, one nonreligious factor was the activism of people living with HIV. There were many turning points where strong activism had an effect, going way back to the beginning of the epidemic. And the activists kept at it. I think it was really very important, especially when HIV and AIDS faded from public consciousness. So, Joost, Olivia, I'm glad you want to give credit to religious leaders, but I think you and WHN and CEAA and your fellow activists can also take some credit here.

Mr. De Jong
Thank you.

Dr. Thomas
Here's something else that isn't religious: scientific data about what works and what doesn't work. For example, the data showed that abstinence-only prevention programs didn't work, but we still pushed them for much too long. And we also knew that mass distribution of condoms didn't work either. Eventually, we realized we needed to push comprehensive prevention programs. Those found their way into the education and empowerment programs. And we've mentioned needle-exchange programs. Data showed they helped prevent HIV transmission, and we rolled them out. Or data about the link between gender-based violence and HIV transmission. Or criminalization. We knew that criminalization of same-sex behavior led to higher rates of HIV transmission. It took us a long time to accept what the data showed, that trying to enforce certain kinds of behavior made the epidemic worse rather than better. But eventually we did, and we began to roll out these programs on a relatively widespread basis.

Rev. Morgan
And an important part of those programs was that they were genuinely comprehensive, including options that had been controversial in the past, such as the use of condoms or the benefits of reducing the number of sexual partners.

Amb. Rogers

You know, I think one other nonreligious motivator was that people gradually began to realize that the boundaries between the marginalized and the rest of society are not impervious. AIDS and HIV thrived among the marginalized. And, for a while, the rest of society could be content, thinking that they were safe because there was a boundary between them and the marginalized. But the margins aren't as solid as we thought. Sex workers have clients who have other sex partners. Women who have been raped hope to lead normal family lives. Recovering injection drug users are trying to fit back into society. Men who have sex with men may sometimes have sex with women. Once we began to realize that HIV could jump across the boundaries, we began to realize that we needed to do something about it.

Dr. Bennett

We saw that same realization gradually growing in the 2010s in the U.S. Two examples. One was the increasing acceptance of the LGBTQ community. There was still a lot of discomfort, but as more and more people came out, many people realized that they had friends and family members who were gay or lesbian, which broke down those marginalization barriers. The other example was the link between HIV infection and the opioid epidemic, which was especially problematic in communities where people never thought that AIDS would be an issue for them. So again, people realized that the boundaries between mainstream and marginalized weren't quite as strong as they had thought.

Dr. Zhang

Thank you.

Now I think it's time to move on to the next topic.

How Important Was Religion in the Global AIDS Response?

Dr. Zhang

Religion has been a controversial part of the AIDS story since the very beginning. Let's talk about that.

Rev. Morgan

May I start? Let's make sure we all remember that faith-based institutions have been part of the global AIDS response from the very beginning. We were out there taking care of people long before there was any kind of treatment, and we're still out there. There have been studies during the entire fifty years of the epidemic. They have consistently shown that between twenty and forty percent of all HIV services are provided by faith-based institutions.

And there are two reasons for this. One is that we are compelled by our faith—we have an obligation to help the sick. The second is that we are pretty much everywhere. Do you remember Rick Warren of Saddleback Church in California? He was part of a big AIDS push by American evangelical churches in the late 2000s. He used to show a slide with a map of Rwanda with all of the medical clinics. There were a few, kind of scattered around the country. And then he showed a slide with all of the churches. The map was

Mr. Joost De Jong:
Religion was, and is, a vital part of our victory over AIDS. If religion hadn't become the strongly positive force that it became, then we wouldn't be sitting here talking about winning the war against AIDS.

---

completely covered. His point was that faith communities have substantial organizational structures that they took advantage of in the AIDS epidemic.

And, of course, the services we provide are available to anybody. We don't care how they got sick. We are just there to take care of them.

Dr. Zhang
What do you say, Joost? Is Emily right?

Mr. De Jong
Yes, she's right. Churches and other faith-based institutions have done a tremendous job of providing HIV services. Nobody is arguing against that. But that's not where the damage was done. The damage was done with respect to the social issues that we just talked about. The stigma we talked about was largely driven by religion. Religious leaders kept pushing these notions that AIDS was God's punishment for bad behavior.

Rev. Morgan
Wait a minute, Joost. There was some of that in the beginning, but it didn't last long.

Mr. De Jong

Well, actually, it lasted a couple of decades at least, so it was pretty important. And even when those leaders stopped talking about God's punishment, they still kept emphasizing all of those so-called "bad" behaviors. That created a lot of stigma.

Imam Karume

You know, stigma is more complicated than that. It's not just a single issue. Let me give you an example. I attended a meeting in Nairobi maybe twelve or fifteen years ago. It was a dialogue between faith leaders and people living with HIV. Stigma obviously came up a lot in the dialogue. But I was really struck by the way that stigma depended on behavior. There was a big difference between stigma toward young people who have premarital sex and stigma toward men who have sex with men. It wasn't just degrees of difference. They were completely different attitudes. Somehow, we could deal with premarital sex, but, in our culture, sex between men was just too far out of the norm for us to even talk about it.

Dr. Bennett

We had different kinds of stigma in the U.S. too. For us, AIDS was initially seen as a gay disease, and that initial perception lasted for a very long time. So, if a woman became infected with HIV, there was always a question, "Wait? What happened here? How did she get it?" She was stigmatized.

Imam Karume

I remember one other thing from the Nairobi meeting. There were both Muslims and Christians, and attitudes about stigma were pretty similar between the two traditions. But we also had some

Rev. Emily Morgan:
I think a large part of the success involved local faith leaders and communities. Many of them actually did a pretty good job at dignity and respect, at providing counseling and support, at not judging, at not stigmatizing.

---

data that showed that stigma was higher in the predominantly Muslim areas. On the other hand, rates of HIV prevalence were still relatively low in the Muslim areas. Fortunately, we were able to defuse the stigma issue and prevent what might have become a big increase in new infections in the Muslim areas.

Dr. Okafor

When we talk about religion and stigma, we need to remember that one of the purposes of religion is to promote good behavior. There will be differences among different religions, like Christianity and Islam. But, in any case, it is basically a moral code, guidance about how people ought to behave. And it's good to have guidelines like that. We want to promote good behavior. But there's a fundamental problem: how can you promote a moral code, any moral code, without somehow stigmatizing people who don't follow it?

Let's separate two different issues. One is: what's the right moral code? The other is: how do you promote a moral code without stigmatizing? Now we're certainly not going to agree on the first issue. Arguments about the right moral code have been going on for millennia, and they'll keep going on for more millennia. But what about the second issue? How do you promote a moral code without stigmatizing? Here is where I fault a lot of religious groups and leaders, especially during the early years of the epidemic. They just weren't very good at treating everybody with dignity and respect.

Whenever somebody disagreed with the moral code, or behaved badly according to the moral code, many religious leaders were very quick to judge.

But then something happened, I'd say it was during the 2010s. Something changed. Somehow religious leaders weren't quite so quick to judge. They acknowledged the differences but treated people respectfully despite the differences. The result was a lot less stigma, the key populations didn't feel so marginalized, and more people were able to get HIV services without fear.

Mr. De Jong

Yes, that's the thing I wanted to say earlier. I used to be strongly anti-religious, and I think I was right to feel that way. But about ten or fifteen years ago, I started having more and more conversations with religious leaders. They just wanted to talk, and soon I saw a whole different side, and I saw more action on their part, and suddenly the barriers were breaking down. We can't underestimate how important that was. On this panel, we were just talking about how important the social issues are and how they got resolved. Well, during the past ten or fifteen years, religious leaders and communities were an indispensable part of resolving those social issues. Religion was, and is, a vital part of our victory over AIDS. If religion hadn't become the strongly positive force that it became, then we wouldn't be sitting here talking about winning the war against AIDS.

Dr. Bennett

Yes, I think most of us would agree with you. It's funny, but initially, there was a widespread perception that religion was part of the problem. And, frankly, to a large degree that perception was justified. But, over time, both the reality and perception have changed. Now, religion is clearly part of the solution.

Dr. Zhang

So, there was a change. What brought about the change?

Rev. Morgan

I think a large part of it involved local faith leaders and communities. Many of them actually did a pretty good job at dignity and respect, at providing counseling and support, at not judging, at not stigmatizing. They worked hard at it. They had specific programs aimed at eliminating stigma.

Imam Karume

Yes, they did. And I think the reason was that they recognized the reality of the AIDS epidemic in their congregations. They saw people dying. They were holding lots of funerals, sometimes several per day. They realized that they had to do something. And they did.

Rev. Morgan

Yes, Ahmed, I'm pretty sure you're right. But it's hard to know when that shift happened. It might have been the late 2000s, or the 2010s. I wish we had had more data about what local faith communities were doing. We had lots of anecdotal evidence about the benefit of programs to reduce stigma in faith communities, but we didn't actually know how many local faith communities were doing what. How many were helping, and how many were hurting? Then somebody did a nice study maybe nine or ten years ago. They identified some criteria to distinguish between faith communities that were actively increasing stigma and faith communities that were actively decreasing stigma. Then they did surveys in several African countries, trying to come up with the percentage of the population that regularly worships at a faith community that increases stigma or decreases stigma. They found that it was an even split, about thirty-five percent each for increasing stigma or decreasing stigma, with the other thirty percent not worshipping regularly. Then they did a similar study a few years later and found that close to sixty percent of the population worshipped at faith communities that helped. That second study showed the dramatic change that we've been talking about, with local faith communities becoming part of the solution, not the problem.

Rev. Morgan

I think one of the reasons for success goes back to that big faith initiative launched by PEPFAR in, what was it? 2018, I think. That initiative helped a lot of local religious leaders and communities deal effectively with the social issues, including stigma. Without that PEPFAR program, we never would have had the good results in that study I mentioned a few minutes ago.

Dr. Bennett

We didn't have any studies like that in the U.S., but we have lots of anecdotal evidence. One thing I noticed was that the 2010s were the period in the U.S. when dialogue between faith leaders and AIDS activists started to pick up steam. For example, many of our CEAA activists were invited to address congregations during worship services.

Imam Karume

There's one other thing that local faith communities did well, especially in Africa. Remember in the 2010s, faith healing became a big deal in many places. Some people living with HIV thought faith healing was a cure, but they died when they stopped taking their medications. Many people died. But then other local faith communities became more aggressive in taking on the faith healers. They worked very hard to make sure that their community members with HIV kept taking their medication. They had things like adherence

Amb. Christopher Rogers:
It was very, very important that prominent global religious leaders spoke out so loudly in the late 2010s and the early 2020s. They were the global conscience that we needed.

---

clubs and support groups. Fortunately, the initiatives eventually overcame the faith healing movement.

Amb. Rogers

There's one other area where I think religion played a vital role: global advocacy.

Rev. Morgan

You know, religious leaders have been global advocates about AIDS for a long time. Think back to Canon Gideon Byamugisha in Uganda. Or the beginning of PEPFAR. Chris, you were at PEPFAR. You know the history. Religious advocacy played a big role in the creation of PEPFAR. President Bush started PEPFAR for moral reasons, not political ones, and many American religious leaders pushed him to do it. And there was a lot of strong advocacy by American evangelicals in the late 2000s. And then, about twenty years ago, UNAIDS organized a meeting with a group of religious leaders. They issued a very strong statement. So religious leaders weren't silent!

Dr. Okafor

Yes, I know. But then there was kind of a quiet period. Do you remember all the marches we used to have at previous AIDS conferences? It always struck me as odd and disappointing that there was barely any participation by religious leaders. There were never more than a few dozen. There should have been hundreds of them! And they should have been at the front instead of hidden in the back.

Amb. Rogers

I had that same feeling too, Chibuzo, all the way through the 2018 conference in Amsterdam. It was so disappointing and frustrating. But then, wasn't it glorious at the San Francisco conference in 2020? Remember there was that summit meeting just before the conference, with some really prominent religious leaders, and then they were the ones that led the march! For me, that march was what marked the transition from religion as a problem to religion as a solution. That's when religious leaders really became the global conscience that we needed, to make sure we all knew that ending AIDS was a moral imperative.

Dr. Zhang

But again, why? Why did all of those leaders suddenly take on such a prominent role? Anybody have any thoughts on that?

Dr. Okafor

I don't know. I'm sure it was a combination of things. I know that there was a lot of soul-searching in the late 2010s, trying to understand the right role for religion in the global AIDS response. I'm sure that the soul-searching was prompted by many different things. For example, in 2016 some aggressive targets had been set for pediatric AIDS, and a lot of energy was put into it, including by a lot of strong religious leaders. But we fell short. That caused a lot of people to ask why.

Rev. Morgan

I know that a lot of religious leaders were really frustrated by the perception that religion was part of the problem, not the solution. I'm sure that was one of the causes of the soul-searching.

Dr. Thomas

I suspect another cause was the growing body of scientific evidence about what worked and what didn't work. It was one of those funny "Science and Religion" discussions. But, in this case, I think it was more about working together than working against each other. As a scientist, I found it rather delightful.

Rev. Morgan

Yes, Jaylen, I'm sure you found it delightful. But I hope you also understand that what worked about those discussions was that you scientists began to recognize that there might actually be some value to religious perspectives.

Dr. Thomas

Yes, you're right. Point taken.

Dr. Okafor

You know, I think we can make a useful comparison with what happened during the Ebola outbreak in western Africa about fifteen years ago. One of the biggest success factors was that community leaders, especially religious leaders, got together and talked about what they needed to do. And then they did it. And Christians and Muslims worked quite well together while they were doing it. I think the fundamental reason was that everybody could see that the Ebola situation was dire and urgent. In the late 2010s, just before the funding slowdown, there wasn't the same sense of urgency about AIDS. But then, the discussions about the Global Fund replenishment in 2019 brought AIDS back to public consciousness, and, suddenly, everybody knew that it actually was urgent. I'll bet that sense of urgency contributed to that soul-searching.

Imam Karume

You know, there's another important point about the Ebola experience. Christians and Muslims were able to work well together. They worked well together because they were focused on solving the Ebola problem. They were so focused on solving an urgent problem that they didn't have time to argue about doctrine or theology. And there was something kind of similar back in the late 2010s. I think it came out of the World Council of Churches. A group of religious AIDS activists—mostly just Christians, but a pretty broad span, including both liberals and conservatives—got together to talk about their differences, and they realized, with respect to ending the AIDS epidemic, that they agreed on almost everything. Their theological and moral differences weren't very consequential if they focused on ending AIDS. And I think that that realization was one of the things that helped in the soul-searching that led up to the San Francisco summit in 2020.

Amb. Rogers

I'd like to mention one other motivator for the soul-searching. I know that many of you were here in Durban for the AIDS conference in 2016. If you were, then I'm sure you remember that amazing speech given by Charlize Theron. It was in this very hall. I went back and found the text of her speech. Her words were quite profound. Here's what she said:

> *The real reason we haven't beaten the epidemic boils down to one simple fact: We value some lives more than others. We value men more than women. Straight love more than gay love. White*

skin more than black skin. The rich more than the poor. Adults more than adolescents.

[Editor's note: At this point, there was prolonged applause, lasting several minutes.]

Dr. Zhang

Yes, that was a great speech, wasn't it? And I know, after that speech, many religious leaders asked themselves, "Is that really true? Do we really value some lives more than others?" I'm sure that was one of the factors that contributed to all of that soul-searching. In any case, whatever led to that soul-searching, I think we can all be glad that it happened.

Let me try to summarize this discussion so we can move on to questions from the audience. Remember, the question before us was: how important was religion in the global AIDS response? Here's what I've heard. First, everybody agrees that religious organizations have done a really good job using their organizational structures to provide HIV services and continue to do so. Second, early in the epidemic, many religious leaders and communities had real difficulty with the complexities of the social issues and actually caused many problems. But then, especially during the past two decades, they got better at it, and now they are a vital partner in addressing those issues. And third, every now and then, religious leaders make a really strong push as global advocates. Two especially important times were early in the 2000s, helping to get PEPFAR launched, and then in 2020, with the summit of religious leaders at the San Francisco AIDS conference.

So, with that, let me bring this topic to a close. I want to make sure we have enough time for questions from the audience.

Questions from the Audience

Dr. Zhang

Now I'd like to open it up to the audience. Please line up at the microphones in the aisles. Well, actually, I can see lines are already forming. Now, you don't need to limit your questions to the three topics we focused on. Your questions can be about anything related to the AIDS epidemic.

Also, I should mention that we have made arrangements with the demonstration leaders to ensure that some of the demonstrators get to ask questions during this session. We've handed out about a half dozen little red cards to some of the demonstrators. As you stand in line, make sure you hold up your red card high so that we can see it from up here.

You first, at microphone number 3. It looks like you have a red card. Please start with your name and where you are from.

Question

My name is Mwenya Banda. My father, Paul Banda, is a Presbyterian minister in eastern Zambia. He is HIV-positive. He went public about his status in 2015, hoping to encourage others to seek testing and treatment. He's been on treatment for a long time, his viral load is suppressed, and he is leading a very productive life, providing spiritual help to hundreds of people. So first, for myself, and on behalf of our congregation, I want to thank you for saving his life. But I would also like to mention something that he often talked about. He liked to make a distinction between moral behavior and safe behavior with respect to AIDS. I think it made a big difference when he helped his congregation understand the distinction.

Imam Karume

I know your father. He is one of the best activists and advocates that we have, full of courage. The distinction you are talking about goes back at least twenty-five years. I first heard it from Rev. Canon Gideon Byamugisha, the founder of INERELA+. He always said that, with respect to HIV and AIDS, we need to distinguish between two dimensions of human behavior. He described them as the "lawful" dimension and the "safe" dimension. In his terminology, he used "lawful" to refer to God's law, so the lawful dimension was behavior that God wanted you to do, like the moral codes we talked about earlier. The safe dimension referred to behavior that does or does not prevent HIV transmission. For the safe dimension, we look to our doctors and scientists for guidance. Gideon's point was that the two dimensions need to be understood and taught differently, but we religious people have a tendency to confuse or mix the two together. We needed to educate people about the distinction. And we needed to make sure that people always followed the safe dimension, even if they didn't always follow the moral dimension.

Dr. Bennett

May I add something? I think that that distinction was part of the reason for the soul-searching that went on among faith leaders in the U.S. During the initial decades of the epidemic, we were often unable to separate the moral and safe dimensions. That's why many of our schools didn't provide enough education about HIV and especially about methods of preventing HIV transmission. But then, in the late 2010s, many American faith leaders began to look at this distinction and realized that failure to make the distinction was one of the root causes of the rise of new HIV infections in the U.S. among young people. As a result, we changed some of our education policies, and new infection rates among young people started to go down again.

Dr. Zhang
Thank you. Next, microphone number 1. I see you also have a red card.

Question
My name is Oksana Silchenko. I come from Russia. I have been married to Andriy for six years. Andriy had been a drug addict before we got married, but I am proud to say that together we have been able to gain control over his addiction. We have recently learned that Andriy was infected by HIV during his addiction years. Fortunately, Andriy was able to get treatment. He now has an undetectable viral load, and I am still HIV negative. We are now able to lead a very normal life, we're planning to have kids, and they'll be fine. I just wanted to thank you. Our lives could have been so much worse. Thank you.

Mr. De Jong
I am glad that you and your husband have his addiction under control. And I appreciate your gratitude, but that wasn't us. It was the Russian government. About ten years ago, they started a much stronger program to combat HIV and AIDS, and you and your husband are a testimony that it worked. Of course, if they had started needle-exchange programs earlier, your husband might not even have become infected with HIV. But we don't need to dwell on that. I'm glad to hear your story.

Dr. Zhang

Thank you. Next, microphone number 2.

Question

My name is Zendaya Moyo. I come from Harare. I just wanted to emphasize what Mr. De Jong said earlier about the effect of viral suppression on self-stigma. I saw that effect. During most of the epidemic, even during the late 2010s, most people living with HIV thought of themselves as failures. But then, as more of them achieved viral suppression, they started feeling more and more hopeful. They saw themselves as real human beings, instead of failures.

Rev. Morgan

Thanks for mentioning that. Yes, I remember. Many of the groups that we worked with were surprised at how quickly people were able to regain their self-respect.

Dr. Zhang

Thank you. Next question, please, you over there at microphone number 3.

Question

My name is Patience Maduka. I come from a rural area in northern Malawi. I am here to thank you on behalf of my cousin Vincent. My aunt, Vincent's mother, was HIV-positive. She was nervous about talking about her status, but her pastor and church friends were very encouraging. She went to the clinic, took her medication, and Vincent was born without HIV. Thank you.

Dr. Thomas

I'm glad to hear stories like this. We've known how to prevent mother-to-child transmission for more than twenty years, but we haven't always been able to fully use that knowledge. There were a few countries that effectively eliminated mother-to-child transmission by the mid 2010s. But then the funding challenges of the late 2010s slowed our progress. We were able to regain momentum by 2021. Fortunately, that was in time for Vincent.

Dr. Zhang
OK, now microphone number 2.

Question
My name is Mary Jefferson. I come from San Angelo, Texas, in the United States. My son Tyler was a star quarterback on his high school football team. Tyler was injured during his senior year and given opioids to relieve the pain. He became addicted and eventually joined a group of young addicts who shared their needles. Fortunately, needle-exchange programs were introduced at about the same time. Without them, I fear that Tyler would have become infected with HIV. So, I just want to thank you that my son is still with us.

Dr. Bennett
I'm very glad to hear about your son. I know that we were slow to roll out needle-exchange programs during the opioid epidemic in the U.S. We knew they worked to prevent HIV transmission, but we were very slow to roll them out. I'm glad we were in time for your son. Of course, there were many others for whom the programs were too little too late.

Dr. Zhang
OK. Microphone number 3, please.

Question

My name is Adila Ahmadi. I live in a village north of Mombasa, Kenya. I remember that a lot of us were confused about HIV and AIDS, especially when it first started to appear in my village. Fortunately, my Imam started an education program and a support program for young people like me. We learned about how HIV spreads and about different ways to avoid getting infected. I believe that what he and the other Imams did was very important in stopping AIDS from becoming a big problem in my village.

Imam Karume

Thank you for sharing your story. I know your Imam, and I know that it was challenging for him and other religious leaders because HIV and AIDS forced us to deal with some pretty complicated issues. I am glad that we were able to overcome the challenge.

Dr. Zhang

OK. Microphone number 2 again.

Question

My name is Ginny Mitchell. I come from the UK. I think you left out one important interaction between religion and AIDS, namely, the influence of religious groups on global political statements. You may remember Sally Smith. She worked at UNAIDS for much of the 2000s and 2010s. In her PhD thesis, she studied the wording of a series of political statements issued at global meetings related to AIDS. I think the statements covered about fifteen years beginning in 2000. She showed that delegations from some countries that were closely aligned with certain religious traditions often pushed hard-line restrictive language. Strong and helpful religious voices got blocked out of the policy debate. As a result, the social issues got much less attention than they deserved.

Dr. Nkosi

I'm glad you mentioned that. I remember Sally's thesis. It's interesting to contrast her results with what happened at the UN High-Level Meeting in 2021, where almost all of the religious input was in favor of a strong commitment to actively addressing the social issues.

Dr. Zhang

Thank you. I'm looking for more red cards. Oh, yes, microphone number 4.

Question

My name is Rodrigo Mendoza. I live in Manila. I am a very active member of my church. In fact, my entire family is very devoted to the church and has been for many generations. Eight years ago, my son, Angelo, learned that he was HIV-positive. He and I talked about it and decided that he should seek advice from our church leaders. We were quite nervous. We didn't know what the leaders would say or do. We had heard old stories about people being thrown out of church. I'm glad to say that our leaders were very supportive, giving us good advice and suggestions about places to get medical help. I want to thank you.

Dr. Okafor

I can't speak for everybody, of course, but you're welcome. Our religious institutions have always been slow to change. I'm glad they changed in time to help your son.

Dr. Zhang

Thank you. Now, microphone number 3.

Question

My name is Michael Robinson. I come from the United States, the state of Indiana. My husband Greg and I got married shortly after same-sex marriage became legal in the United States. He was HIV-positive. We were always careful, and I am still HIV-negative. In the late 2010s, we were quite worried about health insurance, because it looked like HIV might be considered a pre-existing condition and that he would no longer be able to get health insurance. We were both very relieved when the new United States domestic AIDS strategy in 2019 included guarantees that people living with HIV could get insurance.

Dr. Thomas

Well, you know that in the U.S. we had many discussions and arguments about how to provide health care. The big challenge for us was pre-existing conditions. We tried a bunch of different ways to ensure that health insurance was available for people with pre-existing conditions, including HIV. I think we're finally finding more sensible ways to provide health care to everybody, including people with pre-existing conditions. I think that putting together the HIV strategy you mentioned was one of the things that helped us make good progress.

Dr. Zhang

Thank you. I don't see any more red cards. Let's go to you on microphone number 2.

Question

My name is George Michalski. I come from San Francisco. As you look back, what do you think would have happened if the 2019 Global Fund decision had gone the other way? If there had been a reduction instead of an increase?

Dr. Nkosi

Well, there is no doubt that it would have had very serious consequences. I have seen some studies that tried to model different
scenarios. Two things have come out of those studies. First, it would
have been a lot more expensive to regain control of the epidemic. It
would have cost a lot of extra money to catch up if there had been
cuts in 2019. And second, a whole lot of people would have died.
As we mentioned earlier, the studies generally show that between
eight and ten million people would have lost their lives needlessly.

Dr. Zhang

OK. I see one more red card. Microphone number 1.

Question

My name is Lindiwe Ndlovu. I live in Johannesburg. My daughter Thabise was born in 2008. When she was 14, Thabise joined
the DREAMS program, which gave her tremendous support and
encouragement. I had seen what had happened to many young
girls, how they hooked up with Sugar Daddies, became infected
with HIV, and then got dumped. Without DREAMS, I'm sure that
would have happened to Thabise. So, from the bottom of my heart,
thank you for my daughter's life.

Amb. Rogers

I love hearing stories like this. I remember in 2015 when we started
the DREAMS program. It was specifically aimed at young girls
like your daughter. I'm so glad it helped. Thank you for telling us
about her.

Dr. Zhang

Time for one more question. Microphone number 2.

Question

My name is Amanda Stevenson. I come from Chapel Hill, North Carolina, in the U.S. This whole discussion has been very intellectual, very clinical, which is what we would expect from a group of distinguished academics and scientists and doctors. I want to know how you feel. You're sitting up on a stage with a big sign that says, "HOW WE WON THE WAR AGAINST AIDS." How does that make you feel?

Mr. De Jong

For me, it's joy, of course, but also sadness. It's amazing to think we have collectively pulled this off, but I'm also sad for all of those people we lost along the way. I'm sure we could have won the war quicker and better, and then some of those people might still be here with us. But mostly it's joy!

Amb. Rogers

For me, I think it's a feeling of relief. I look back at all of those times and places where we could have gone wrong. And, in fact, I know that there were many things that did go wrong. But, in the end, we did enough things right that we can be up here celebrating. But it was close! I remember back in the late 2010s, we could so easily have given up, or even just slowed down. And then we'd be here on a stage with a sign that says, "HOW WE LOST THE WAR AGAINST AIDS." I can't imagine how depressing that would have been. So, I am really, really relieved to be on a stage with this sign and not the other one.

Dr. Nkosi

I keep thinking about the millions of people whose lives were saved. Every one of those people is a living, breathing, human being, with family and friends and hopes and dreams. They are the ones whose feelings really matter. I just have a sense of satisfaction, maybe even a little bit of gratitude, for having been part of the global effort that gave them lives to lead and feelings to have.

Imam Karume

I know that pride is a dangerous sin, but, in all honesty, I have to admit to feeling a little pride that we religious folk were so instrumental in coping with the social issues. I remember something that a friend of mine once said. Rev. Phumzile Mabizela was the Executive Director of INERELA+ for many years. She once said to me, "If we can't do this..." She was speaking about people of faith dealing with the social issues like stigma. She said, "If we can't do this, what good are we?" Well, we did do it! So we must be worth something after all!

Dr. Zhang

Thank you, Joost, Chris, Munashe, Ahmed.

For me, the really strong feelings go back to that critical period from 2015 to 2020. I remember a feeling of hope back in 2016, when we were last here in Durban. Hope that we really could end AIDS by 2030. But then that hope was replaced by fear at the HIV Science Conference in Paris the next year, when we started to see data showing that the rate of new infections wasn't going down like it needed to. And the dismay and disbelief I felt at the Amsterdam conference, when it looked like things really were slipping away, that the political will was disappearing. I couldn't believe that we would throw away all of the great work that had been done and that we would let HIV and AIDS come back. But then there was that Global Fund meeting in 2019. Suddenly, I felt hope again. The resources were going to be there, and that gave me a feeling of determination. Then there was that great march at the San Francisco conference in 2020, with all of those prominent religious leaders. I'm not a particularly religious person, but that march was really inspiring. And, for the first time, I really believed that we would be able to deal with the social issues because religion would unquestionably be on our side. Then, a few years later, that belief was confirmed when we started getting data about what so many local faith communities were doing. And all of that came out at about the same time that we finally crossed the incidence/prevalence threshold, 0.030, in 2023. At that point, I knew, we all knew, that we would ultimately win, that we wouldn't have to worry about a sign with the word "LOST" in place of the word "WON."

Closing Remarks

Dr. Zhang

Sorry, I got a little long winded with that, but it's probably a good transition into the final part of this panel. Let's close by looking again at the name of the panel, *How We Won the War Against AIDS.* I'd like us to list the most important things that we did well, what mistakes we avoided, and what opportunities we seized. I don't want any rambling comments here. I want something specific, that if it had gone the other way, we might not have won the war. Let's start with you, Ahmed, and then go down the line.

Imam Karume

I am very glad that we put so much effort into educating our young people and into providing safe spaces and support for them during their formative years.

Dr. Nkosi

I am very grateful that the American government provided such strong leadership at the end of the 2010s, not just at the medical and technical level, but at the global political level. Obviously, they had been providing strong leadership for years, but in the last half of the 2010s, there was a real risk that the global response would collapse. American leadership was instrumental in avoiding that collapse.

Mr. De Jong

May I mention two? First, I think that messaging about viral suppression was very important, like that "U=U" campaign fifteen years ago. Campaigns like that really helped people living with HIV overcome self-stigma. Second, it was very important that we found ways to get HIV services, including prevention services, to key populations without risk of criminal prosecution. It wasn't always about changing the laws. The key thing was that we put policies and mechanisms in place that allowed them to get services despite the laws.

Rev. Morgan

I am very glad that so many local religious communities put so much effort into fighting stigma. I wish they had done it earlier, but, ultimately, they came through. And frankly, it helped a lot that we developed ways of measuring what they were doing. The data provided a lot of guidance to local and national religious leaders.

Dr. Okafor

I am pleased that the countries in western Africa recognized the challenges of HIV and AIDS in time to put effective programs in place. That was especially helpful for our young people, preventing the bubble of infections that we feared we would experience in the 2020s. And I am especially gratified that churches and mosques were a central element of the programs for young people.

Dr. Bennett

I am very glad that the United States launched the *Ending the HIV Epidemic* program in 2019 and successfully implemented it along with the other elements of a comprehensive strategy. Many of us were surprised when it was announced, and a bit skeptical, but it actually did happen. That's why we closed down the Campaign to End AIDS in America in 2027—we weren't needed anymore!

Dr. Thomas

It's really good that we finally began to adapt laws and policies to align with scientific evidence, especially about what worked and what didn't work in preventing new infections.

Amb. Rogers

It was very, very important that prominent global religious leaders spoke out so loudly in the late 2010s and the early 2020s. They were the global conscience that we needed.

Dr. Zhang

Thank you.

To close this session, I'd like to quote Charlize Theron again. This is how she ended her speech in 2016:

> *Since the first International AIDS Conference in 1985, we have been counting up, all the way to 21. Now it's time for us to start counting down. We have set a goal to end the AIDS epidemic by 2030. There are seven more International AIDS Conferences between now and then. They must be our last.*

It is such a wonderful feeling to be able to say that we have lived up to the challenge she set for us fourteen years ago. This conference, the 28th International AIDS Conference, is indeed the last. We can all be very proud of winning the war against AIDS. Congratulations!

[Editor's note: At this point, confetti and balloons were released. There was prolonged applause, lasting more than fifteen minutes.]

Charlize Theron (2016)

The real reason we haven't beaten the epidemic boils down to one simple fact: We value some lives more than others. We value men more than women. Straight love more than gay love. White skin more than black skin. The rich more than the poor. Adults more than adolescents.

Dr. Zhang Xiu Ying (2030)

After that speech, many religious leaders asked themselves, "Is that really true? Do we really value some lives more than others?"

Panelists

Olivia Bennett, PhD

Dr. Bennett is on the faculty of Yale University in the School of Public Health. She was formerly the President and Chief Executive Officer of the Campaign to End AIDS in America, a leading AIDS advocacy organization in the United States that operated from 2010 through 2027. Dr. Bennett earned her PhD in Public Policy from the University of Chicago. In 2024, she was named to lead the Campaign to End AIDS in America and served until its board decided to close the organization following the success of the United States' *Ending the HIV Epidemic* program.

Joost De Jong

Mr. De Jong is the Executive Director of WHN, the Worldwide HIV Network. For many years, Mr. De Jong has been a prominent advocate for the human rights of people living with HIV or at risk of HIV infection. He was named the Executive Director of WHN in 2025.

Rafael González, MD

Dr. González is on the faculty of Universidade de São Paulo, where he leads the Medical School Public Hospital. He earned his undergraduate degree at Universidade Federal do Rio de Janeiro and completed his MD at the Universidade de São Paulo in 2009. In 2028, he was elected to serve a two-year term as President of the International AIDS Society. He is the Co-Chair of the 28th International AIDS Conference.

Ahmed Karume, BA

Imam Karume is the Executive Director of INERELA+, the International Network of Religious Leaders Living with or Personally Affected by HIV or AIDS. Imam Karume received his undergraduate degree at Umma University in Kenya and his religious training at the London Muslim Centre. He served numerous congregations in Kenya and then joined the staff of INERELA+ in 2023. He became Executive Director in 2028.

Emily Morgan, MTh, DD

Rev. Morgan is the Executive Director of Christian Health Alliance, an umbrella organization for a number of Christian non-governmental organizations. Rev. Morgan is an ordained pastor. She was educated at the Boston University School of Theology. She served as a health missionary in a variety of countries before joining CHA in 2021. She has been the Executive Director of CHA since 2028.

Munashe Nkosi, MD

Dr. Nkosi is the Executive Director of the Global Fund to Fight AIDS, Tuberculosis and Malaria. She received her medical degree from the University of Cape Town, specializing in Infectious Diseases. She joined WHO in 2006, serving in various positions before moving over to the Global Fund to become Executive Director in 2027.

Chibuzo Okafor, PhD

Dr. Okafor is the Director of African Projects for International

Interfaith Relief Services. He earned his undergraduate degree in Health Sciences at the University of Lagos and a PhD in Public Health from the University of Nigeria. He has served with IIRS for more than twenty years at many locations around the world. He was named Director of Africa Projects in 2027 and is based in Lagos.

Christopher Rogers, MD, PhD
Amb. Rogers was the United States Global AIDS Coordinator and directed the PEPFAR program from 2023 through its closure in 2028. He earned his PhD in International Development from Stanford University. He worked for many years at USAID before returning to Harvard Medical School, where he earned an MD with a specialty in Epidemiology. He joined PEPFAR in 2016 and was selected to lead the agency in 2023.

Jaylen Thomas, MD, PhD
Dr. Thomas is the Director of the Centers for Disease Control and Prevention in the United States. He earned an MD in Primary Care from Columbia University and then a PhD in Public Health from Johns Hopkins University. He served for many years at UNAIDS and WHO before being named the Director of the CDC in 2022.

Zhang Xiu Ying, PhD
Dr. Zhang is the Director-General of the World Health Organization. She earned her undergraduate degree at Tsinghua University and her PhD from the University of Oxford, with a specialization in International Health Policy. During her twenty-year career, she has worked for numerous international health organizations. She was selected to lead the Global Fund to Fight AIDS, Tuberculosis and Malaria in 2026.

"How We Won the War Against AIDS"
Recorded by SA Media Consultants
Durban, South Africa
29 July 2030

Afterword

I hope this is a work of nonfiction, but it might not be. The AIDS epidemic is at a tipping point. If we tip in the right direction, we will have a future like the one depicted in this transcript of a future panel at a future AIDS conference. Unfortunately, a bright future is not inevitable. If we fail to do what we know how to do, we will have a future like the one depicted in the other half of this book, a transcript from a future panel titled *How We Lost the War Against AIDS.*

> David R. Barstow
> June 2019
> Corvallis, Oregon, USA

It Is Not 2030, It Is Only 2019 …

If the trends continue through the decade of the 2030s, there will be many more needless new infections and needless deaths ...

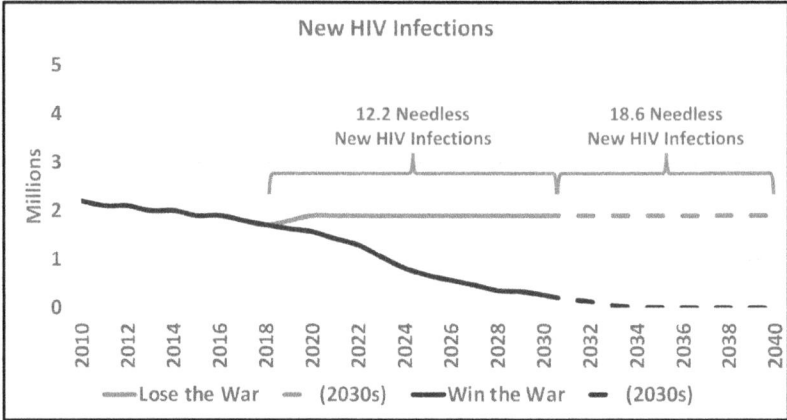

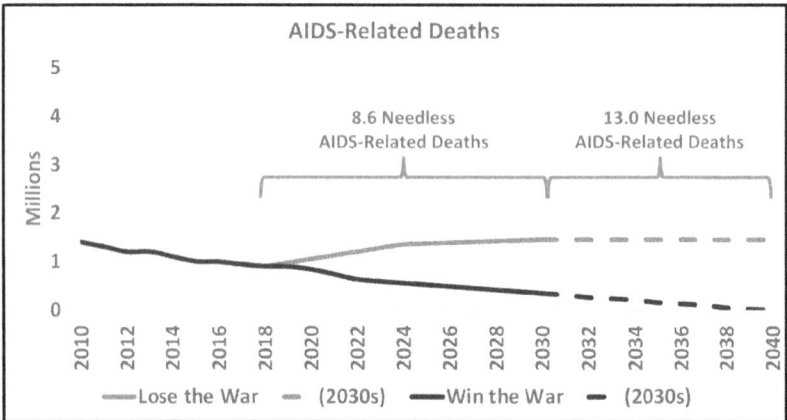

New HIV Infections

12.2 Needless
New HIV Infections

18.6 Needless
New HIV Infections

Millions

5
4
3
2
1
0

2010 2012 2014 2016 2018 2020 2022 2024 2026 2028 2030 2032 2034 2036 2038 2040

Lose the War — (2030s) Win the War — (2030s)

AIDS-Related Deaths

8.6 Needless
AIDS-Related Deaths

13.0 Needless
AIDS-Related Deaths

Millions

5
4
3
2
1
0

2010 2012 2014 2016 2018 2020 2022 2024 2026 2028 2030 2032 2034 2036 2038 2040

Lose the War — (2030s) Win the War — (2030s)

Choosing the Future

One way or the other, 2030 will be a year of reckoning for the global response to the AIDS epidemic. But, of course, it is now only 2019. We don't yet know which future we will see in 2030, which form that reckoning will take. We don't yet know whether we will win or lose the war against AIDS.

The differences between the two futures are stark. In the losing future, 12.2 million more people become infected with HIV, and 8.6 million more people die than in the winning future. And that is only through 2030. In the winning future, both new infections and deaths are low in 2030 and heading even lower. In the losing future, both numbers have stabilized and are likely to continue at similar levels for many more years. If the trends continue through the decade of the 2030s, we could have an additional fifteen to twenty million needless new infections and an additional ten to fifteen million needless deaths, with no end in sight.

Fortunately, in 2019, it is still within our collective power to avoid that prospect. We can still win the war against AIDS, and we can take some suggestions about how to do that from comments made by the experts on both imaginary future panels.

With respect to funding, several important decisions will be made in 2019. The Global Fund replenishment meeting in Lyon will be critical. We must collectively decide to increase the amount in the Global Fund by at least the 15% requested in the investment case. American leadership would go a long way toward ensuring that this decision is made. At the same time, it is also critically important that recipient countries commit to a significant increase in their share of the costs of battling AIDS within their boundaries, and they must ensure that funds are used effectively.

With respect to the United States domestic battle against AIDS, the critical decisions will be those concerned with allocating funds for the strategy developed in early 2019, as mentioned by President Donald Trump in his State of the Union address. That announcement was met with a certain amount of surprise and skepticism by American AIDS activists. The proof will be in the allocation of funds to support the strategy, including not only the *Ending the HIV Epidemic* program, but also other elements of the American health care system, such as the widespread availability of HIV testing, treatment, and prevention services.

But funding decisions are not enough to win the war against AIDS. If funding decisions go the wrong way, we will surely lose. But simply going the right way on funding decisions doesn't guarantee victory. We must also navigate the complexities of the social issues. HIV and AIDS thrive among the marginalized, and we must find ways to bridge the boundaries that separate the marginalized from the rest of society. We must ensure that HIV treatment services are available to all people living with HIV, and we must ensure that HIV prevention services are available to key and vulnerable populations that are at increased risk of infection. We must provide these services without judgment, stigma, discrimination, or risk of criminal prosecution.

Empowering young people is critically important to ending AIDS. We must accept that young people face many challenges during their formative years, and we must equip them to deal with those challenges. This will be especially important in some of the high-burden areas of Africa and elsewhere, which risk a sudden rise in new HIV infections among young people. And it will also be important in the United States, where too often our young people are not educated about HIV and other sexually transmitted diseases and are not equipped with full knowledge about prevention options.

Whereas we can identify certain specific funding decisions that are make-or-break for the global response to the AIDS epidemic, success with the social issues will require many small decisions about services and policies in many regions for many years. In situations where these decisions are controversial, we must look to scientific evidence for guidance on which programs to implement, always with the long-term objective of ending the AIDS epidemic.

I, for one, don't see how we can successfully navigate the social complexities of the AIDS epidemic without the active involvement of religious leaders, communities, and institutions. Religion was the most controversial topic addressed by the future expert panelists. Both panels identified ways in which religion had significantly helped and significantly hurt the global response to the AIDS epidemic. Religion was both a part of the problem and a part of the solution. In the "losing" panel, the mixture of problem and solution continued through 2030. In the "winning" panel, there was a significant change in the late 2010s, highlighted by a global summit of religious leaders in 2020, after which religion was unquestionably an active part of the solution.

There may or may not be a summit of religious leaders in San Francisco next year, but the panelists identified several other ways in which religion could strengthen its role in the AIDS epidemic, so that it becomes unquestionably part of the solution. One way is advocacy. Prominent religious leaders could strengthen their voices, stressing the moral imperative of ending the AIDS epidemic and the urgency of acting strongly before it is too late. For example, religious leaders could be especially influential in the funding decisions to be made in 2019 about the replenishment of the Global Fund and about appropriations for the United States domestic HIV plan.

But, perhaps more importantly, religious leaders and communities are a vital part of the solution at the local level. Many studies have shown that high percentages of the population of high-burden countries attend worship services regularly. The future panelists noted several ways that those places of worship could play a very strong role in addressing the social issues related to HIV and AIDS—for example, by reducing stigma and judgmental attitudes, by helping people living with HIV adhere to their medical treatment, by helping to educate and empower young people, by reducing gender-based violence, and by reaching out to the marginalized. If such activities are undertaken by large numbers of places of worship in high-burden countries, we will go a long way toward successfully addressing the social complexities of the AIDS epidemic.

It is not 2030. It is 2019. It is not too late to choose the future.

Future and Present Perspectives

The future panelists are all looking back at fifty years of HIV and AIDS. From their perspective, everything they say refers to their past and their present. Of course, from our perspective in 2019, some of the things they say are in the future.

Data in the epidemiology and investment charts are historically accurate through 2017. For example, much of the data comes from the UNAIDS website. Information on the charts for 2018 through 2030 were created to illustrate the two futures. The charts are generally consistent with other models and projections but should not be interpreted as precise projections of the future.[1]

Places and events with dates before 2018 are historically accurate. For example, two of the conferences in the series of International AIDS Conferences have been held in Durban, South Africa, once in 2000 and once in 2016. The next International AIDS Conference will be held in 2020 in San Francisco. However, there are, as yet, no plans for a summit of prominent religious leaders to be held at the same time as the conference. There was a special session of the United Nations General Assembly in June 2001. There was a High-Level Meeting on AIDS at the United Nations in September 2016. There was a Global Fund replenishment meeting in September

1. For more details about other models and projections, see "Data and Modeling" on page 162.

2016. There will be a replenishment meeting in Lyon, France, in October 2019. There have been many meetings to promote dialogue between religious leaders and people living with HIV, including one in Nairobi, Kenya, in February 2017.

People identified before 2018 are real people. Charlize Theron, the actor from South Africa, gave an inspiring speech at the 2016 conference. Dr. Jonathan Mann led the first AIDS initiative of the World Health Organization. Dr. Peter Piot referred to "two possible futures" in a speech to the special session of the General Assembly of the United Nations in June 2001. Dr. Sally Smith formerly worked at UNAIDS and wrote a PhD thesis on the influence of religion on various political declarations related to HIV and AIDS.[2] Rev. Canon Gideon Byamugisha is an Anglican priest in Uganda who was open about being HIV-positive in the 1990s and who founded INERELA+. Rev. Phumzile Mabizela, the current Executive Director of INERELA+, once said to me, "If we can't do this, what good are we?"

All of the future panelists are imagined. Some of them work for real organizations, including PEPFAR, the World Health Organiza-tion, The Global Fund to Fight AIDS, Tuberculosis and Malaria, the Centers for Disease Control and Prevention, and INERELA+. Other organizations, such as Worldwide HIV Network, International Inter-faith Relief Services, Christian Health Alliance, and the Campaign to End AIDS in America, have been invented, but they are intended to be representative of the types of organizations that are currently active in the domestic or global response to HIV and AIDS.

Most of the initiatives mentioned by the panelists are real. In 2019, the United States Government announced a new program

2.   Smith, Sally. 2018. *Religion in the United Nations (UN) Political Declarations on HIV/AIDS: An Interdisciplinary, Critical Discourse Analysis.* Doctor of Practical Theology, Theology and Religious Studies, School of Critical Studies, Glasgow. http://theses.gla. ac.uk/30615/13/2018smithdpt.pdf

called *Ending the HIV Epidemic*, intended to significantly reduce new HIV infections in the United States. In 2018, PEPFAR announced a major initiative to support faith-based organizations in the global fight against AIDS. In 2015, PEPFAR launched the DREAMS initiative focused on helping girls and young women in sub-Saharan Africa. The HOPES initiative, focused on helping boys and young men, as described by Rev. Morgan, is imagined. However, there have been increased efforts to engage men more fully in the AIDS response. For example, the MenStar coalition, including many of the major global AIDS organizations, was launched in 2018.

In a few cases, some of the panelists make statements about the past that are not fully supported by data. For example, Rev. Morgan says that between twenty and forty percent of HIV services are provided by faith-based institutions. However, there are not sufficient data to either support or refute her remark.[3] That is why panelists in both futures talk about the importance of gathering much more data about the actions taken by faith-based institutions and by local faith communities in response to HIV and AIDS.

All of the future audience participants are imagined. They are intended to be representative of the millions of people around the world who are affected by HIV and AIDS.

But what really matters in 2019 is our present perspective, not that of future panelists. In our past, we have already made remarkable progress in the war against AIDS, both globally and domestically in the United States. In our present, we are making choices and taking actions that will determine our future—whether we win or lose the war against AIDS.

---

3.   For more information about academic studies of the religious response to AIDS, see "Religion and AIDS" on page 171.

Appendix:
Background Information

HIV and AIDS

HIV

Human Immunodeficiency Virus is a virus that attacks the human immune system. Untreated, the virus slowly weakens the immune system over the course of several years. During the early stages of the disease, a person with HIV may not have any apparent symptoms.

AIDS

Acquired Immunodeficiency Syndrome is an advanced stage of HIV infection. A person with AIDS may develop a variety of opportunistic infections and other diseases. Untreated, a person with AIDS typically survives for no more than three years.

Treatment

Infection with HIV is no longer a death sentence. It is a manageable chronic condition. Treatment with antiretroviral drugs (ARVs) stops the progression of the disease and ultimately leads to a condition known as viral suppression in which HIV is still present but not detectable.

There is presently no cure for HIV. Scientists are actively working to develop a cure, but it will be many years before an effective cure is available. To date, two patients have been cured in the process of receiving bone marrow transplants as a treatment for cancer, but the process is very risky and expensive and therefore not reliable or scalable.[4]

---

4. "H.I.V. is reported cured in a second patient, a milestone in the global AIDS epidemic," *New York Times*, March 4, 2019. http://www.nytimes.com/2019/03/04/health/aids-cure-london-patient.html

Prevention

HIV is transmitted from one person to another through the exchange of certain bodily fluids, most commonly through sexual activity, but HIV can also be transmitted through blood transfusions, shared syringes, or from a mother to her child through pregnancy, birth, or breastfeeding. A variety of prevention methods are available with varying degrees of effectiveness. Generally speaking, a combination of methods offers the best chance to prevent transmission.

Treatment itself constitutes a strong form of prevention. A person who has achieved viral suppression through ARV treatment is extremely unlikely to transmit the virus to another person.[5]

There is presently no vaccine to protect against HIV. Clinical trials of several vaccine candidates are underway. A partially effective vaccine is a possibility in the next five to ten years.

5.   Alison J Rodger, et al. "Risk of HIV transmission through condomless sex in serodifferent gay couples with the HIV-positive partner taking suppressive antiretroviral therapy (PARTNER): Final results of a multicentre, prospective, observational study," *The Lancet,* May 2, 2019. http://www.thelancet.com/journals/lancet/article/PIIS0140-6736(19)30418-0/fulltext

History of the AIDS Epidemic

Early 1900s

The most recent analysis is that HIV was first transmitted to human beings from monkeys somewhere in western Africa in the late 1800s or early 1900s.[6] It spread slowly in Africa for many decades.

1980s

AIDS first gained significant public attention in the United States in the 1980s as the disease spread rapidly in several cities among men who had sex with men. The disease also began to appear among Haitians, probably through guest workers who had been brought back from Africa after colonial rule was over.[7]

In 1984, HIV was identified as the virus that causes AIDS.

1990s

During the 1990s, HIV spread very rapidly in eastern and southern Africa, reaching a peak rate of 3.5 million new infections in 1995.[8] Prevention programs, such as large-scale public information campaigns, began to reduce the rate of new infections in some countries.

In 1995, ARV therapy first became available as a treatment for HIV and AIDS. It rapidly came into use in the late 1990s in upper-income countries like the United States, but the treatment was too expensive for widespread use in lower- and middle-income countries.

6. For a discussion of the origins of HIV, see "Origins of HIV & AIDS" on the Avert website: http://www.avert.org/professionals/history-hiv-aids/origin

7. "H.I.V. arrived in the U.S. long before 'Patient Zero,'" *New York Times,* October 26, 2016. http://www.nytimes.com/2016/10/27/health/hiv-patient-zero-genetic-analysis.html

8. Unless otherwise indicated, all epidemiological data in this section are taken from the UNAIDS website: http://aidsinfo.unaids.org/

UNAIDS, the primary United Nations agency dealing with HIV and AIDS, was created in 1996, followed by significant efforts to mobilize the world community to fight the disease.[9]

2000s

Major international initiatives were launched in the early 2000s to stop the growing humanitarian catastrophe. A special session of the United Nations General Assembly met in 2001 and issued a Declaration of Commitment on HIV/AIDS. The Global Fund to Fight AIDS, Tuberculosis and Malaria was launched in 2002, providing a mechanism by which wealthier countries could assist poorer countries to address the three diseases. In 2003, the United States launched PEPFAR, the President's Emergency Plan for AIDS Relief, significantly increasing both the funding and the technical capacity available to fight AIDS globally. PEPFAR and the Global Fund were largely responsible for the rapid rollout of ARV treatment in the high-burden countries of Africa. By 2010, 7.6 million people were on ARV treatment.

As part of the global rollout, the ARV treatment protocols have become much simpler, and the cost of routine ARV treatment has gone down dramatically. During the 2000s, thanks to the availability of generic versions, the average annual cost per person in sub-Saharan Africa went from more than $10,000 to less than $100.[10]

The rates of new infection, which had peaked at 3.5 million in 1995, continued to decline, reaching 2.2 million in 2010. The rates of

9.   Piot, Peter. 2012. *No Time To Lose: A Life in Pursuit of Deadly Viruses.* New York: W. W. Norton & Company. http://books.wwnorton.com/books/No-Time-to-Lose/

10. "HIV treatment now reaching more than 6 million people in sub-Saharan Africa." UNAIDS, July 6, 2012. http://www.unaids.org/en/resources/presscentre/pressreleaseandstatementarchive/2012july/20120706prafricatreatment

AIDS-related deaths peaked in 2005 at 1.9 million, but then began to decline, reaching 1.5 million in 2010.

2010s

The rates of new infections and AIDS-related deaths continued to decline in the 2010s. Figure A-1 on page 156 shows the numbers of new HIV infections and AIDS-related deaths during the first thirty-seven years of the epidemic.

The availability of ARV treatment spread rapidly during the 2010s. As shown in Figure A-2 on page 156, the number of people receiving treatment reached 20 million by 2017.

During the 2010s, there were growing numbers of HIV infections related to injection drug use. For example, Russia experienced a significant increase in new HIV infections, primarily due to transmission among people who use drugs.[11] In the United States, there has been a growth of new HIV infections associated with the opioid epidemic.[12]

During the 2010s, there was also a significant increase in the fraction of the financial cost that was carried by the high-burden countries themselves. By 2017, domestic sources accounted for 56% of the funding, the Global Fund accounted for 10%, U.S. bilateral sources such as PEPFAR accounted for 25%, and other international sources accounted for 9%.[13]

11. Cohen, Jon. "Russia's HIV/AIDS epidemic is getting worse, not better," *Science,* June 11, 2018. http://www.sciencemag.org/news/2018/06/russia-s-hivaids-epidemic-getting-worse-not-better

12. Dawson, Lindsey, and Jennifer Kates. "HIV and the Opioid Epidemic: 5 Key Points." Henry J. Kaiser Family Foundation, March 27, 2018. http://www.kff.org/hivaids/issue-brief/hiv-and-the-opioid-epidemic-5-key-points/

13. UNAIDS website: http://hivfinancial.unaids.org/

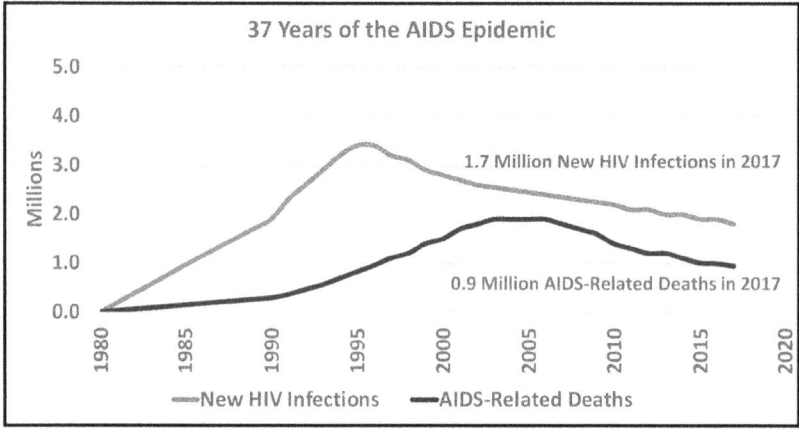

Figure A-1—Thirty-Seven Years of the AIDS Epidemic

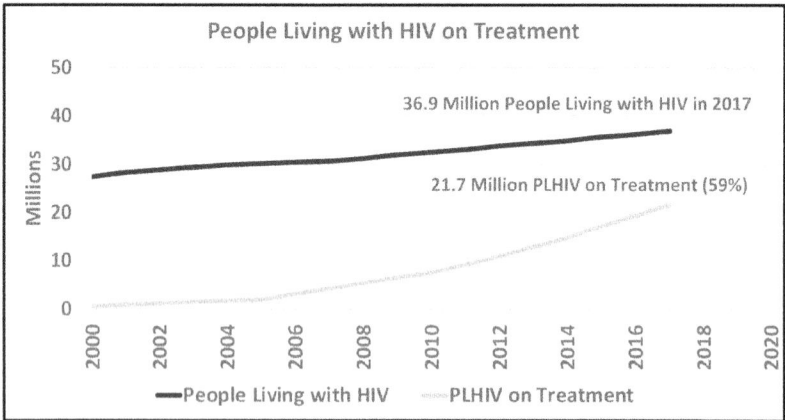

Figure A-2—People Living with HIV on Treatment

Current State and Future Risks

Global AIDS Epidemic

HIV prevalence is defined to be the percentage of the population that is infected by HIV. Figure A-3 on page 158 shows the HIV prevalence rates for adults by country, as of the end of 2017.[14]

HIV incidence is defined to be the number of new infections by HIV within a population. Figure A-4 on page 158 shows the HIV incidence rates per 1,000 people by country, as of the end of 2017.

Future Risks

However, despite all of the remarkable progress, there are indications that HIV and AIDS are not yet under control and might make a comeback in the 2020s. The greatest concerns are related to new infections. The number of new infections has not gone down as quickly as expected, and there is a significant risk of a rapid increase in new infections among young people in high-burden countries.

On World AIDS Day, December 1, 2014, UNAIDS launched its Fast Track strategy intended to finally bring the epidemic under control and to end HIV and AIDS as public health threats by 2030.[15] The Fast Track targets were expressed in terms of the HIV treatment cascade. The targets for 2020 are:

90% of the people who have HIV know their status

90% of the people who know their status are on treatment

90% of the people on treatment have suppressed viral load

---

14. This map, and the map of new HIV infections worldwide, are taken from the UNAIDS website: http://aidsinfo.unaids.org/

15. "Fast-Track strategy to end the AIDS epidemic by 2030." UNAIDS, December 1, 2014. http://www.unaids.org/en/resources/campaigns/World-AIDS-Day-Report-2014

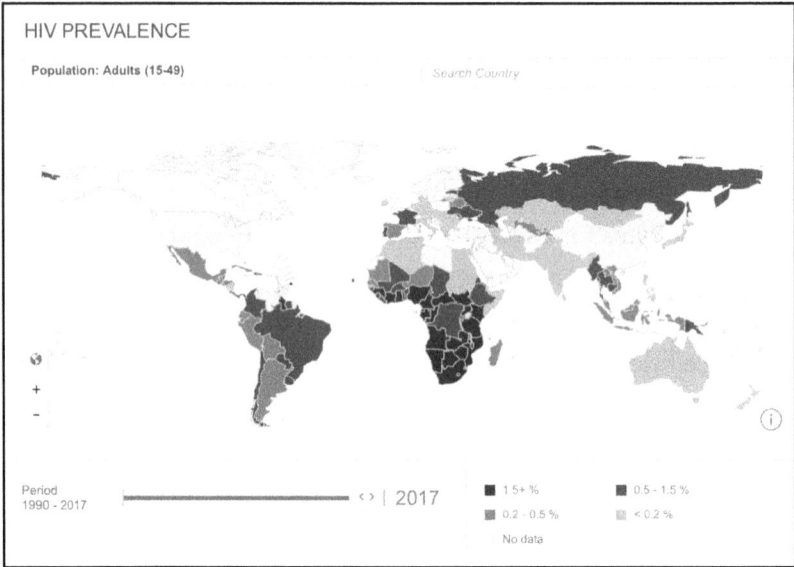

Figure A-3—HIV Prevalance (Worldwide)

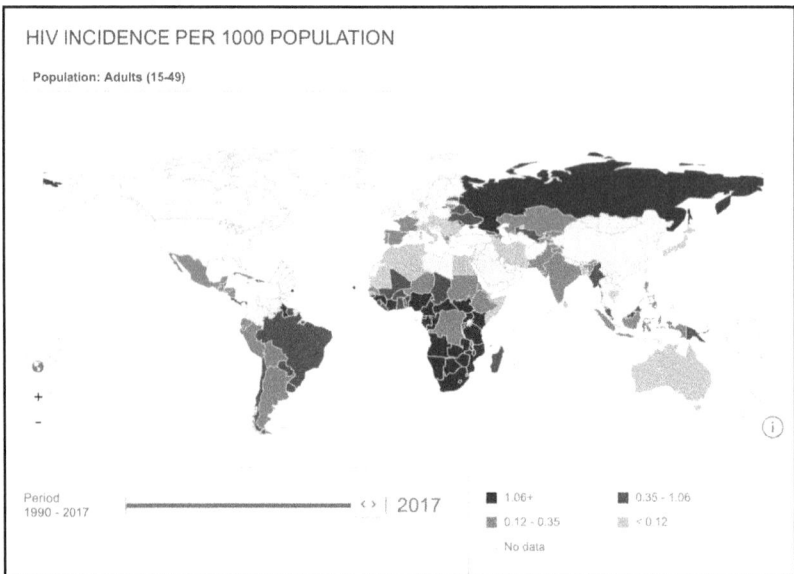

Figure A-4—HIV Incidence (Worldwide)

As of early 2019, it seems unlikely that these targets will be met in 2020. Different countries are having different degrees of success. Some are on track to achieve 90-90-90, but globally the targets seem out of reach. The table below shows the progress through the end of 2017, the latest year for which data are available.[16]

Measure	Millions	Percentage of PLHIV	Percentage by Stage
People with HIV	36.9		
People who know their status	27.5	74.5%	74.5%
People who are on treatment	21.7	58.8%	78.9%
People with suppressed viral load	17.5	47.4%	80.6%

AIDS in the United States

There are currently about 1.1 million people in the United States who are living with HIV. Each year, there are about 38,500 new HIV infections and 6,000 AIDS-related deaths.[17]

The table on page 160 shows the treatment cascade numbers for the United States.

16. Treatment cascade data are taken from the UNAIDS website: http://aidsinfo.unaids.org/
17. Data about the AIDS epidemic in the United States are taken from the government's HIV website: http://www.hiv.gov/hiv-basics/overview/data-and-trends/statistics

Measure	Millions	Percentage of PLHIV	Percentage by Stage
People with HIV	1.1		
People who know their status	0.95	86%	86%
People who are on treatment	0.69	63%	73%
People with suppressed viral load	0.56	51%	81%

Among people living with HIV in the United States, young people were the most likely to be unaware of their status.

Figure A-5 on page 161 shows the rate of new HIV diagnoses in the United States by state in 2015, that is, the number of people newly diagnosed with HIV per 100,000 people. Although not identical, the rate of new HIV diagnoses correlates closely to HIV incidence.[18]

The map illustrates changing trends in the AIDS epidemic in the United States. In 2015, more than half of the new HIV diagnoses were in the south.

18. This map is taken from the website of the Centers for Disease Control and Prevention: http://www.cdc.gov/hiv/statistics/overview/geographicdistribution.html

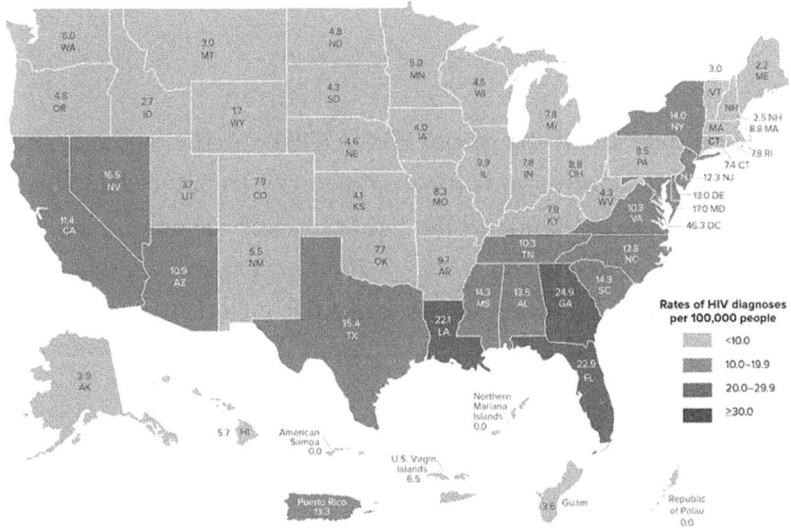

A-5—New HIV Diagnoses (United States)

Data and Modeling

Data Sources

Detailed data about the global HIV/AIDS epidemic are available
from UNAIDS (http://aidsinfo.unaids.org/). Detailed data about
the HIV/AIDS epidemic in the United States are available from
the CDC (http://www.cdc.gov/hiv/statistics). Other comprehensive
sources of information about HIV and AIDS include AVERT (http://
www.avert.org/) and the Kaiser Family Foundation (http://www.
kff.org/hivaids).

Modeling and Projections

Detailed epidemiological and investment models about the HIV
and AIDS epidemic have been developed and used to project future
trends and to inform public policy decisions. UNAIDS' Fast Track
strategy, launched in 2014, was based on modeling that compared
two future scenarios. One scenario showed that constant levels
of funding would lead to a resurgence of the epidemic. The other
scenario showed that HIV and AIDS could be eliminated as threats
to public health by 2030 with increased levels of funding. Models
are periodically updated and adapted to reflect the passage of time
and the availability of new information. Some of the key modeling groups are Avenir Health (http://www.avenirhealth.org/), the
UNAIDS Reference Group on Estimates, Modelling and Projections
(http://www.epidem.org/), and the HIV Modelling Consortium
(http://www.hivmodelling.org/).

Charts of the Two Futures

The fifty-year charts used in the transcripts of this book were created
to illustrate the differences between two divergent futures, as seen
from a 2030 perspective. They are generally consistent with other

models, but they should not be interpreted as precise projections of the future from a 2019 perspective.

The charts are based on data from several sources, including actual data about the epidemic through 2017 from UNAIDS,[19] the original Fast Track and Constant Coverage models developed in 2014,[20] projections done by John Stover of Avenir Health in early 2018 to reflect the effects of a cut in funding,[21] and the 2019 Global Fund replenishment case.[22]

19. UNAIDS: http://hivfinancial.unaids.org/; http://aidsinfo.unaids.org/

20. Stover, John, et al. "What is required to end the AIDS epidemic as a public health threat by 2030? The cost and impact of the fast track approach," *PLOS ONE,* May 9, 2016. http://journals.plos.org/plosone/article/figure?id=10.1371/journal.pone.0154893.g001

21. Stover, John, personal communications.

22. "Step Up the Fight." The Global Fund to Fight AIDS, Tuberculosis and Malaria, March 7, 2019. http://www.theglobalfund.org/en/stepupthefight

Treatment Cascade

HIV Status

The HIV status of a person is either HIV-positive or HIV-negative. HIV-positive means that the person has been infected by HIV. HIV-negative means that the person has not been infected by HIV. Since there is no cure for HIV infection, a person who is HIV-positive will remain HIV-positive for life, although some tests might be negative due to successful treatment. Many people are HIV-positive but are not aware of their status. There are a variety of tests to determine a person's HIV status, although some tests may show false negative due to successful treatment.

HIV Treatment

The current WHO guidelines for HIV treatment suggest that a person be put on ARV medication as soon as they know they are HIV-positive. HIV treatment involves a rigorous protocol, including regular tests for the effectiveness of the treatment. The treatment protocols have become simpler over time, and now generally involve a single pill containing a drug cocktail, once per day. For a variety of reasons, many people who know that they are HIV-positive may not be on treatment, and many people who are on treatment may not follow the protocol or may abandon treatment completely.

Viral Suppression

When HIV treatment protocols are followed, a person's viral load, that is, the amount of HIV present in the body, will gradually decline. Ultimately, a person will reach a state of viral suppression in which HIV is no longer detectable, although it is still present in the body. Once viral suppression is achieved, a person must continue following the treatment protocol in order to remain virally suppressed. A person with suppressed viral load is extremely unlikely to transmit HIV to another person.

Combination Prevention

HIV Transmission

HIV is transmitted from one person to another through the exchange of certain bodily fluids that contain large concentrations of HIV, specifically, blood, semen, vaginal and rectal secretions, and breast milk. Other bodily fluids, such as sweat, tears, and saliva, do not contain large concentrations of HIV, so they can be exchanged without risk of HIV transmission. This means, in particular, that HIV cannot be transmitted through casual contact.

Modes of Transmission

The most common mode of HIV transmission is through sexual contact. As outlined below, there are many options available for avoiding the risk of HIV transmission through sexual activity.

Another common form of HIV transmission is from a mother to her child, either during pregnancy, birth, or breast feeding. ARV treatment for the mother during and after pregnancy generally prevents this mode of transmission. By ensuring that all pregnant mothers receive treatment, many countries have effectively eliminated mother-to-child transmission.

In the early years of the epidemic, HIV was sometimes transmitted through blood transfusions. However, this mode of transmission is now extremely rare, since blood used for transfusions is routinely screened for the presence of HIV.

Another common mode of transmission is through sharing of needles used by people who inject drugs. Needle exchange programs, as well as other harm-reduction strategies, have proven effective at reducing the risk of this mode of HIV transmission.

Prevention Options

There are a variety of options for preventing the transmission of HIV. Some are related to specific modes of transmission. For sexual transmission, the options include use of a condom, medical male circumcision, and reduction in the number of sexual partners.[23] For mother-to-child transmission, ARV treatment during and after pregnancy is very effective. For HIV transmission by shared needles, the best option is simply not to share needles, which can be facilitated by needle exchange programs.

Other prevention options apply to all modes of transmission. For example, pre-exposure prophylaxis (PrEP, a daily pill) prevents an HIV-negative person from being infected by HIV. Similarly, if an HIV-positive person has achieved viral suppression, that person cannot transmit the disease to another person, except under very rare circumstances.

It is not always possible to prevent HIV transmission. For example, a victim of gender-based violence may become infected by HIV in a situation in which the victim has no control. Likewise, an accidental prick by an infected needle can also lead to HIV infection.

Prevention Programs

It is important that organized prevention programs employ strategies and policies that include the full range of prevention options, guided by the needs of different key and vulnerable populations. Strong prevention programs also address underlying social drivers that increase the risk of HIV transmission, such as gender-based violence and addiction to injection drugs.

23. "What can decrease HIV risk?" Centers for Disease Control and Prevention. http://wwwn.cdc.gov/hivrisk/decreased_risk/

Social Drivers

Key Populations

For a variety of reasons, there is a significantly greater risk of HIV infection among certain groups of people, including men who have sex with men, people who inject drugs, people in prisons and other closed settings, sex workers, and transgender people. One risk factor is that members of these groups may engage in behavior with increased risk of HIV transmission, such as unprotected sexual activity or sharing of syringes. Another risk factor is that these groups are often marginalized by society, which makes it more difficult for them to access HIV prevention and treatment services.

Vulnerable Populations

Other groups of people are at increased risk in some settings, including women and girls, children and adolescents, and migrant and mobile workers. The increased risk is often due to the relatively weak position that these groups may hold in society. For example, where women and girls have a low social status, they are especially vulnerable to gender-based violence, which in turn can lead to HIV infection. Women and girls also have an increased biological vulnerability to HIV infection.

Stigma

Stigma is a judgmental attitude toward individuals or groups perceived to be different. Stigma associated with HIV and AIDS is the result of several factors. One factor is simply fear of contracting the disease by associating with someone who is HIV-positive. Another factor, perhaps more important, is that HIV infection is often associated with behavior that is perceived to be bad by mainstream society. There may be different degrees of stigma, depending on how bad the behavior is perceived to be. For example, stigma toward people engaged in extramarital sex may be quite different from stigma toward men who have sex with men, and both might be different from stigma toward people who inject drugs.

Stigma toward people living with HIV is a significant barrier to ending AIDS because fear of stigma often stops people from getting tested and treated. They are afraid of rejection by family and community. Stigma also makes it more difficult for members of key and vulnerable populations at risk of HIV infection to access HIV prevention services. Finally, stigma often leads to loss of self-respect by the stigmatized persons, making them less likely to access HIV prevention and treatment services.

Discrimination

Whereas stigma is an attitude, discrimination involves policies and behavior that treat people living with HIV differently from those without HIV. Discrimination may be subtle, such as avoiding people known or suspected of having HIV. Discrimination may be overt, such as treating people differently at a medical clinic or restricting travel. Discrimination may have significant economic implications, such as termination of employment.

Fear of discrimination adds to the fears already felt by a person with HIV, making it even more challenging to access HIV testing and treatment services.

Criminalization

Some countries have laws against some of the behaviors of members of key populations. For example, many countries have laws against same-sex relationships, sex work, or the use of injection drugs. While the merits of these laws may be debated, they are certainly a barrier to accessing HIV prevention and treatment services. A person is much less likely to seek services when faced with the possibility of criminal prosecution and imprisonment.

Societal Forces

In addition to the social drivers related directly to HIV and AIDS, there are also societal forces that exacerbate the complexities of dealing with all diseases, including HIV and AIDS, such as racism, poverty, malnutrition, unsanitary water supplies, and weak health delivery systems.

Scientific Studies

Two good collections of scientific studies about the effects of stigma on the HIV epidemic were published by *The Lancet* in 2014 ("HIV: Science and stigma," *The Lancet*, July 19, 2014. http://www. thelancet.com/journals/lancet/article/PIIS0140-6736(14)61193-4) and by STRIVE, a research consortium organized by the London School of Hygiene & Tropical Medicine, in 2019 (http://strive.lshtm.ac.uk/).

Religion and AIDS

HIV Services

Religious organizations and institutions have played a prominent role in providing HIV and AIDS services since the beginning of the epidemic. In many countries, faith-based clinics and hospitals are an integral part of the public health system. Local faith communities are often involved on the front lines, since they may be much more accessible than other public health facilities. In addition, many religious traditions have large relief and development organizations that are substantially involved in providing HIV and AIDS services.

Moral Dilemmas

One role of religion is to provide guidance about how to lead a good life. Different religions, of course, promote different guidelines, and even within a religious tradition, guidelines may sometimes seem to work at cross purposes. This is clearly seen in the AIDS epidemic, for example, when members of some religious traditions are strongly motivated by compassion to help the sick by providing HIV services, even though the context involves behavior that they view as morally wrong. As a result, many religious leaders and communities have had difficulty dealing with the social drivers that have such a strong effect on the AIDS epidemic.

Influence on Public Policy

Religion can have a significant role in the formation of public policy. For example, religious leaders played a vital role in the development of PEPFAR, motivated largely by compassionate and humanitarian concerns. On the other hand, some religious leaders have also argued strongly for restrictive laws, for example, against same-sex behavior, despite the fact that such laws make it harder to fight the AIDS epidemic. The underlying challenge is a fear that some elements of public health policy that may help stem the AIDS epidemic may also encourage behavior that violates a religious tradition's moral guidance. As of 2019, this underlying challenge hasn't yet been resolved to widespread satisfaction.

Advocacy

Many religious traditions include activism and advocacy about issues of social justice. In the context of the AIDS epidemic, this may take many forms, including advocacy for the human rights of key and vulnerable populations, for universal availability of HIV services, and for the repeal of laws that hinder the response to HIV and AIDS.

Local Religious Communities

In many areas, local religious leaders and communities have a significant influence, not only on their members but also on the wider community. For example, studies of countries in sub-Saharan Africa generally show that 80% or more of the population attend weekly worship services. In other regions, the rates are lower. For example, in the United States the rate of weekly attendance is only 36%.[24]

In countries with high rates of attendance, there is great potential for local religious leaders to have a significant influence on the local AIDS response. Indeed, a great many religious leaders in Africa have made very significant contributions to the AIDS response in their communities. However, there is much less data about how widespread such contributions are. As of 2019, we don't know how broadly the potential influence of religious communities on the local AIDS response is being realized.

24. "How religious commitment varies by country among people of all ages." Pew Research Center, June 2018. http://www.pewforum.org/2018/06/13/how-religious-commitment-varies-by-country-among-people-of-all-ages/

Interreligious AIDS Initiatives

Many religious AIDS initiatives have found strength in working across the boundaries between religious traditions. For example, for many years, the Ecumenical Advocacy Alliance, now an initiative within the World Council of Churches, has organized an Interfaith Pre-Conference at the site of the biennial International AIDS Conferences (http://www.oikoumene.org/en/what-we-do/eaa/faith-on-the-fast-track).

INERELA+, the International Network of Religious Leaders Living with or Personally Affected by HIV or AIDS, has members from a broad range of religious traditions (http://www.inerela.org/).

The Common Voice initiative was launched in 2018 to provide a broadly interreligious platform for advocacy and action to end AIDS (http://www.commonvoiceaids.org/).

ACHAP, the African Christian Health Associations Platform, recently released a counseling guide for religious leaders that includes contributions from Muslims as well as Christians (http://africachap.org/wp-content/uploads/2019/04/HIV-and-AIDS-Guide.pdf).

For More Information

A recent issue of the *American Journal of Public Health* contained a number of articles about the role of religion in public health, including the HIV epidemic (Alfredo Morabia, "Faith-based organizations and public health: Another facet of the public health dialogue," *American Journal of Public Health*, February 6, 2019. http://ajph.aphapublications.org/doi/10.2105/AJPH.2018.304935).

The Lancet has published a series of articles about the role of religion in medicine ("Faith-based health care," *The Lancet,* July 7, 2015. http://www.thelancet.com/series/faith-based-health-care).

In addition to these two collections, the following articles provide good summaries of what is currently known about the religious response to HIV and AIDS:

Olivier, J., C. Tsimpo, R. Gemignani, et al. "Understanding the roles of faith-based health-care providers in Africa: Review of the evidence with a focus on magnitude, reach, cost, and satisfaction," *The Lancet*, October 2015. (http://www.thelancet.com/journals/lancet/article/PIIS0140-6736(15)60251-3/fulltext)

Olivier, Jill, and Sally Smith. "Innovative faith-community responses to HIV and AIDS: Summative lessons from over two decades of work," *The Review of Faith and International Affairs*, September 2016. (http://www.tandfonline.com/doi/full/10.1080/15570274.2016.1215839)

Blevins, John. "Are faith-based organizations assets or hindrances for adolescents living with HIV? They're both," *Brown Journal of World Affairs*. (http://bjwa.brown.edu/22-2/are-faith-based-organizations-assets-or-hindrances-for-adolescents-living-with-hiv-they-are-both/)

Coleman, Jason D., Allan D. Tate, Bambi Gaddist, and Jacob White. "Social determinants of HIV-related stigma in faith-based organizations," *American Journal of Public Health*, March 2016. (http://ajph.aphapublications.org/doi/full/10.2105/AJPH.2015.302985)

Activism

People Living with HIV

Activism by people living with HIV has been an important driver of the global response to HIV and AIDS since the beginning of the epidemic. One of the first was ACT UP, the AIDS Coalition to Unleash Power, founded in New York City in 1987 (http://actupny.com/). TAC, the Treatment Action Campaign, was founded in South Africa in 1998 (http://tac.org.za/). GNP+, the Global Network of People Living with HIV, was officially founded in 1992, with roots going back to 1986 (http://www.gnpplus.net/).

GIPA and MIPA

One of the guiding principles of the global AIDS response is that people living with HIV should be actively and meaningfully involved in shaping the response. The principle was first articulated at a conference in Denver in 1983 (http://vpwas.com/gipa-mipa-and-the-denver-principles/). The acronym GIPA, Greater Involvement of People Living with HIV/AIDS, was first used at the Paris AIDS Conference in 1994. Since then, it has evolved to become MIPA, Meaningful Involvement of People Living with HIV/AIDS. The principle includes two parts:

1. To recognize the important contribution people living with HIV can make in the response to the epidemic, and
2. To create space within society for PLHIV involvement and active participation in all aspects of that response.

International AIDS Candlelight Memorial

The International AIDS Candlelight Memorial is held annually on the third Sunday in May. It is organized by GNP+ to both remember those who have died from AIDS-related diseases in the previous year and to raise awareness and to mobilize the AIDS community (http://www.candlelightmemorial.org/). Its roots go back to 1983, when four men in San Francisco started a candlelight march that soon grew to include thousands of people.

World AIDS Day

December 1 is internationally recognized as World AIDS Day, a day to focus global attention on an epidemic that has killed more than thirty-five million people and that has not yet been brought under control (http://www.worldaidsday.org).

Organizations

International Organizations

UNAIDS (Joint United Nations Programme on HIV/AIDS) is the primary United Nations agency for dealing with the HIV and AIDS epidemic (http://www.unaids.org/).

The **Global Fund for AIDS, Tuberculosis and Malaria** is the primary mechanism for high-income countries to provide financial support to help low-income countries fight the three epidemics (http://www.theglobalfund.org/).

WHO (World Health Organization), the primary international organization dealing with global health issues, has a department focused on HIV and AIDS (http://www.who.int/hiv).

The **International AIDS Society** is the largest scientific organization devoted to the study of HIV and AIDS (http://www.iasociety.org/). The IAS organizes a major conference each year. In odd-numbered years, the conference is referred to as the **IAS Conference on HIV Science.** It will be held in Mexico City in 2019 (http://www.ias2019.org/). In even-numbered years, the conference has a broader scope and is referred to as the **International AIDS Conference.** The 2020 conference will be in San Francisco (http://www.aids2020.org/).

United States Government

PEPFAR (President's Emergency Plan for AIDS Relief) is the primary United States agency for dealing with the global HIV/AIDS epidemic (http://www.pepfar.gov/).

The United States government has several agencies dealing with various aspects of the domestic HIV/AIDS epidemic, including

the **Centers for Disease Control and Prevention** (http://www.
cdc.gov/hiv) and the **National Institutes of Health** (http://www.
nih.gov/research-training/hiv/aids-info-center). In early 2019, the
U.S. government announced a new domestic HIV/AIDS initiative
referred to as *Ending the HIV Epidemic* (http://www.hiv.gov/).

Non-Governmental Organizations

There are many thousands of non-governmental organizations and
foundations that are devoting significant effort to winning the war
against AIDS. The following list is necessarily very incomplete, but
I hope it is representative and useful.

The **Bill and Melinda Gates Foundation** is a major non-governmental contributor to the global AIDS response (http://www.
gatesfoundation.org/What-We-Do/Global-Health/HIV).

The **Clinton Foundation,** through the Clinton Health Access
Initiative, was instrumental in reducing the cost of HIV treatment
in low-income countries (http://www.clintonfoundation.org/our-
work/clinton-health-access-initiative).

amfAR (American Foundation for AIDS Research) supports a
broad range of research activities (http://www.amfar.org/).

The **Kaiser Family Foundation** is engaged in the fight against
HIV and AIDS on many fronts (http://www.kff.org/hivaids/).

The **Elizabeth Glaser Pediatric AIDS Foundation** supports
a broad range of activities focused on children and young people
affected by HIV or AIDS (http://www.pedaids.org/).

The **Elizabeth Taylor AIDS Foundation** supports a broad range
of organizations that provide services to people living with HIV or
AIDS (http://www.elizabethtayloraidsfoundation.org).

The **Elton John AIDS Foundation** funds frontline activities
providing HIV services to people living with HIV and at risk of
HIV infection (http://www.ejaf.org/).

The **Charlize Theron Africa Outreach Project** is focused on empowering young people in Africa to prevent a surge in HIV infections (http://www.charlizeafricaoutreach.org/).

ONE is a large international advocacy organization with a major initiative focused on HIV and AIDS (http://www.one.org/). ONE works closely with an affiliated program known as **(RED)** that partners with companies who commit a portion of their revenue from specific products to support HIV and AIDS treatment and prevention programs (http://www.red.org/).

Other American HIV/AIDS advocacy groups include **TAG** (Treatment Action Group, http://www.treatmentactiongroup.org/), **AIDS United** (http://www.aidsunited.org/), and **NMAC** (http://www.nmac.org/). NMAC organizes the **United States Conference on AIDS**, held annually in early September (http://2019usca.org).

Faith-Based Organizations

The list of faith-based organizations that have played important roles in addressing the HIV and AIDS epidemic is much too long to include here, so I can only list a few that I have had the good fortune to work with.

The **World Council of Churches** has two initiatives devoted to HIV and AIDS, **WCC-EHAIA** (Ecumenical HIV and AIDS Initiatives and Advocacy, http://www.oikoumene.org/en/what-we-do/ehaia) and **WCC-EAA** (Ecumenical Advocacy Alliance, http://www.oikoumene.org/en/what-we-do/eaa/faith-on-the-fast-track). **CABSA** (Christian AIDS Bureau of Southern Africa, http://www.cabsa.org.za) provides resources and training to help Christian communities address the HIV and AIDS epidemic. **CCIH** (Christian Connections for International Health, http://www.ccih.org) is an umbrella organization for a number of Christian NGOs. **World Vision**, an international Christian relief, development, and advocacy organization, works closely with local community faith leaders in fighting HIV and Ebola (World Vision US, http://www.worldvision.org/; World Vision International, http://www.wvi.org/church-and-interfaith-engagement/channels-hope-hiv).

Within the United States, the **USCA Faith Coalition** organizes a pre-conference in coordination with the United States Conference on AIDS (http://www.ucc.org/uscafaith). The **National Faith-Based HIV/AIDS Awareness Day** is held every year in late August (http://faithaidsday.com).

As a member of the Presbyterian Church (USA), I have worked closely with the **Presbyterian World Mission** team (http://www.presbyterianmission.org/ministries/world-mission/) and with its Zambia, Zimbabwe, Mozambique Mission Network. The **Presbyterian AIDS Network** (http://www.presbyterianmission.org/ministries/ phewa/pan/) is active within the United States.

Acknowledgments

Jonathan Quick and David Robinson have been vital partners in the development of this book. I met them both for the first time in June 2018 at the annual conference of Christian Connections for International Health. Jono and I gave a tag-team presentation about the role of religion in fighting epidemics, with a focus on HIV and AIDS. Immediately afterwards, Dave spoke passionately with us about the importance of the message. They have both worked hard with me for the past year to help shape the book and to help spread the message.

John Stover of Avenir Health has been very helpful in developing the charts used by the future panelists. He helped me understand the complexities of quantitative models and projections of the future of epidemics. I appreciate his advice and suggestions.

The book has benefited greatly from colleagues who have read and commented on earlier versions, including Mona Bormet, Ulysses Burley, Chris Collins, Doug Fountain, George Kerr, Mark Lagon, Francesca Merico, Martha Ndlovu-Teijema, Bob Noziglia, Lyn van Rooyen, Anita Smith, Sally Smith, and Shepherd Smith.

I appreciate the help of Teresa Welch of Wild Iris Communications and Sheridan McCarthy and Stanton Nelson of Meadowlark Publishing Services, who helped ensure the professional quality of the book.

I also appreciate the feedback from my fellow writers in Lill Ahrens' group at the Writers Ready Room, including Cristy Brickell, Shriya Inuzuka, Ruth McNeill, Kathie O'Brien, Sue Ploeger, Dana Schaffer, Barbara Schultz, and Janice Woodard.

Thanks also to my friends in the Friday afternoon discussion group at Imagine Coffee House in Corvallis who have encouraged me throughout this project, including Roger Blaine, Dick Clinton, Dick Colley, Ron Hershel, David Rabinovitz, Jim Rawers, Megha Shyam, and Dick Weinman.

I first had the idea of looking back from a point in the future of the AIDS epidemic in July 2016, after some discussions at the 21st International AIDS Conference in Durban. The first incarnation of the idea was a video produced in Austin, Texas, in the summer of 2017, which I like to describe as the trailer for a documentary film that will be made in 2030 (http://www.vimeo.com/waragainstaids/trailer). Many thanks to a great group of people who helped produce the video, including Mario Mattei, who directed the production; Rich Terry, who helped with the script; and Jamie Jennings, who edited the final result. Hanna Cofer and Molly von Berg helped with our online presence and social media.

Last year, I coordinated the Common Voice team, developing a way to talk about the HIV and AIDS epidemic that would be consistent across a broad range of religious traditions (http://www. commonvoiceaids.org/). Many people made substantial contributions to the initiative, including Kadhija Abdullah, Seth Christopher Yaw Appiah, Father Rick Bauer, Dionne Boissiere, Ulysses Burley, Rev. Canon Gideon Byamugisha, Prof. Ruard Ganzevoort, Christo Greyling, Rev. Neelley Hicks, Dan Irvine, Manuella Kalsky, Flavia Kyomukama, Rev. Phumzile Mabizela, Marsha Martin, Francesca Merico, Marianne Moyaert, Martha Ndlovu-Teijema, Rev. Edwin Sanders, Rev. Mike Schuenemeyer, Anita Smith, Sally Smith, Shepherd Smith, and Carl Stecker. The video was produced with the help of David and Olivia Giglio of Skyline Video Productions and David Hausen and his team from Surreel Films.

During my dozen years as an AIDS activist, I have been blessed to spend time with many remarkable people, in addition to those I have already mentioned. With apologies to those whose names are not here because of my fading memory, the list includes: Maria Abernathy, Miles Abernathy, Katy Ajer, Bill Alloway, Mary Alloway, D. T. Banda, Pearson Banda, Phil Barnes, Victoria Barrera, Joy Barstow, Vicky Barstow, Astrid Berner-Rodoreda, Willem Bester, Yvonne Bester, John Blevins, Amy Bloomquist, Larry Bloomquist, David Bock, Paul Bonde, Rebekah Bonde, Bono, Debbie Braaksma, Susan Bright, David Bryden, Beverly Chasse, Anne Child, Kingsley Chirwa, Joseph Collins, Nancy Collins, Eric Crabtree, Suzy Denner, Lloyd Doggett, John Doty, Rebecca Duerst, Sharon Edwards, Gloria Ekpo, Kathy Erb, Mike Ervin, Judy Ervin, Karen Farabee, Sally Findley, Doug Fletcher, Ruth Foley, Aneleh Fourie-le Roux, Carol Friesen, Paul Friesen, Bill Galloway, Rosemary Galloway, Allan Gerson, Matt Gough, Andy Greenawalt, Peggy Greenawalt, Janet Guyer, Jan Tore Hall, Ruthann Hall, Pete Hayes, Ron Herschel, Sally Hilderbrand, Susan Hillis, Regan Hofmann, Mike Hogan, Van Hoisington, Nomfuse Hude, Karen Hughes, Stacy Ikard, Charles Johnson, Melissa Johnson, Paul Keith, Susie Kelly, George Kerr, Mimi Kiser, Jimmy Kolker, Sandy Kress, Al Krummenacher, Manoj Kurian, Christine Lambden, Tom LaSalvia, Anya Malkov, Barbara Malloy, Buyelma Maringa, Barbara Martinson, Keith Martinson, Andisiwe Matiwane, Rosemary Matsikidze, Beth McGrath, Jesse Milan, J. P. Mokgethi-Heath, Teboho Motumi, Minnie Moyo, Buhle Mpofu, Debra Mwale, Costen Mwale, Meman Mwandila, Jane N'gan'ga, Steve Neville, Nyambura Njoroge, David North, Linda North, Laura Nyblade, Stanley Nyirenda, Tom O'Meara, Sue Perry, Gerald Phiri, Isabel Phiri, Karen Plater, Mark Ramsey, Tim Roach, Lyn van Rooyen, Lisa le Roux, Fred Shaub, June Shaub, Karen

Sichenga, Gretchen Singh, Sara Speicher, Tami Schroeder, Ryan Smith, Laurel Sprague, Anne Stangl, Joyce Statz, Doug Tilton, Janet Tobias, Jacek Tyszko, Pamella Vakala, Bob Vitillo, Alan Washington, Ted Wright, and Ginger Zanetti. Many thanks to each of you for all you have done and shared.

Finally, but very far from least, I want to thank my family: my parents, Robbins and Meg Barstow, for setting such good examples of social activism; my siblings and siblings-in-law, Cedar Barstow, Dan Barstow, Reynold Feldman, and Eva Barstow, for their encouragement; my son and daughter and their families, Geoff Barstow, Suzie Cooper, Eliza Barstow, Meg Barstow, and Daniel Cooper, for their love; and especially my wife, Linda, who has loved me and supported me and shared in this new calling that pushed our life in an unplanned, sometimes uncomfortable, but always gratifying direction.

About the Author

David R. Barstow is a computer scientist turned AIDS activist. After earning his PhD in Artificial Intelligence from Stanford University in 1977, David spent the next thirty years as a college professor, industrial research scientist and engineer, internet entrepreneur, and business consultant. A remark by Bono, the Irish rock star, at a 2006 Christian leadership conference prompted him to change directions. Since then, David has focused his time and energy on strengthening the religious response to the AIDS epidemic. In 2007, he founded EMPACT Africa, a Christian non-profit dedicated to working with local faith leaders in southern Africa to address the stigma associated with HIV and AIDS. During the past decade, he has worked with numerous governmental, non-governmental, and faith-based organizations. Most recently, David worked with the World Council of Churches to coordinate the Common Voice initiative, an interreligious movement of advocacy and action to end AIDS.

www.ingramcontent.com/pod-product-compliance
Lightning Source LLC
Chambersburg PA
CBHW060319030426
42336CB00011B/1119